Take This Book to the **Obstetrician** with You

A CONSUMER'S GUIDE TO PREGNANCY AND CHILDBIRTH

Karla Morales and Charles B. Inlander

Addison-Wesley Publishing Company, Inc.

Reading, Massachusetts   Menlo Park, California   New York
Don Mills, Ontario   Wokingham, England   Amsterdam   Bonn
Sydney   Singapore   Tokyo   Madrid   San Juan
Paris   Seoul   Milan   Mexico City   Taipei

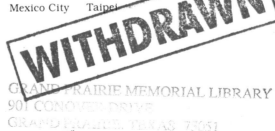

Library of Congress Cataloging-in-Publication Data

Morales, Karla.
   Take this book to the obstetrician with you : a consumer's guide
to pregnancy and childbirth / Karla Morales and Charles B. Inlander.
     p.   cm.
   "A People's Medical Society book."
   Includes index.
   ISBN 0-201-52380-9
   1. Pregnancy. 2. Childbirth. 3. Consumer education.
I. Inlander, Charles B. II. Title.
RG525.M574   1991   90-27768
518.2—dc20   CIP

Cover design by Hannus Design Associates
Text design by Jennie Bush, Designworks, Inc.
Set in 10-point ITC Bookman by DEKR Corporation, Woburn MA

1 2 3 4 5 6 7 8 9-MA-9594939291
First printing, May 1991

Contents

Preface

Obstetrics, as a medical specialty, is a rather recent phenomenon. In fact, the medicalization of childbearing is relatively new. Only in this century have the overwhelming majority of births been attended by physicians. In the United States, it was not until after World War II that more babies were born under doctors' eyes than under those of a midwife or other lay attendant.

Hospitals also are new to the birthing scene. Prior to the 1940s more people were born at home than in a facility. The surprising fact that there has been only one United States president—Jimmy Carter—born in a hospital vividly underscores the point.

Today's high-tech world of gizmos, gadgets, bells, and whistles has transformed what was once a natural event into a medical diagnosis, an almost-disease. What used to be an experience overseen by family, friends, and neighbors is now supervised, and often controlled, by specially trained doctors and nurses, many of whom live in fear that their patients' expectations of their competence may result in a debilitating lawsuit if all does not go as planned.

The medicalization of childbirth has had a chilling effect on consumers. Many women feel helpless in the presence of their doctors. Obstetricians often speak a language rooted in Latin, Greek, or technospeak. Electrodes and cold metal instruments have replaced hands and warm words of encouragement.

Paying for childbirth with a doctor has become a package deal. It is not unusual for a certain number of visits, a variety of scans and tests, and an uncomplicated delivery to be offered for one prearranged price. And, of course, there is another package price for the "complicated" delivery that might include a cesarean section. Although there are certainly advantages to package pricing, it underscores the impersonal and businesslike nature of what was traditionally a warm, family-centered experience.

The women's health movement has been one bright ray of sanity and force in this otherwise medically invasive picture. Since the mid-1970s, hospitals have modified their maternity services to meet the market: a female population that has demanded change. Some obstetricians have changed their practice patterns to make them more forthcoming and accessible, and accepted greater participation by the delivering woman and her partner in the pregnancy and birth.

Even with these changes, however, every woman contemplating having a child is confronted with an enormous array of issues and hundreds of decisions to be made. And in order to face these issues and make the choices, she must be informed and empowered.

Empowerment is taking control of one's own situation. Empowerment is having the information necessary to assure that the way you go through your childbirth experience is your way. Like the old commercial slogan, "Have it your way . . . Have it your way," childbirth should be your way, the way you want it to be—under your control, with you making the ultimate decisions.

Take This Book to the Obstetrician with You is designed to put you in control. It is quite different from other pregnancy books. Our goal is to help you cut through the red tape, and understand what you will be confronted with and how you can be in charge every step of the way. From infertility to surrogacy, midwives to high-risk obstetricians, prenatal to neonatal procedures—here are the pros and cons of just about everything you will encounter.

- Should you have your baby at home?
- What about cesarean sections? What can you do to prevent a first one or a repeat?
- Does your obstetrician have experience with a particular problem you might have?
- What about all the available tests? Are some safer than others? Is your age a factor in tests?
- What should you know about the hospital you plan to use?

These issues (and much more) are covered.

What makes this book unique is our concern that you and your baby have the experience most appropriate to your needs and wishes. We are not trying to push any specific method of treatment, or any particular type of practitioner or setting. We have reviewed and studied the medical literature. We have talked to experts in all the relevant disciplines. We have approached this book with a completely open mind about what is appropriate or inappropriate care. And we have done something else that you will not find in most other books about pregnancy and childbirth: we have left out anecdotes. This book is based on factual data, not stories. We made sure our sources were legitimate and supportable. While another individual's experience may make for a good read, it does not necessarily provide you with the valid information you need to make a decision.

That is what empowerment is all about. It is having valid information on which you can make a decision. When you are finished reading this book, you will have the tools to be an empowered consumer of obstetrical services. Your pregnancy and childbirth experiences will be smoother, not because we have given you all the answers, but because we have shown you the questions you must ask—and why you should ask them.

The empowered consumer receives the best care, gets the best service, and usually has the best outcome. Obstetricians and other medical professionals know that people who ask questions play an active role in their care and demand respect and consideration.

Since our founding in 1983, hundreds of thousands of medical consumers have used the People's Medical Society as their guide through the medical maze. As America's largest consumer health advocacy organization, we are committed to helping you have it your way.

Having a child should be one of the most exciting events in a woman's life. Nothing that can be avoided should get in the way of making it just that. *Take This Book to the Obstetrician with You* is your companion, your tool, to ensure that throughout the entire process you are in charge.

Charles B. Inlander
President
People's Medical Society

Acknowledgments

Too often, authors receive sole credit for what is truly a collaborative effort. In this case, many individuals and organizations helped produce what is now before you.

Nancy Miller, our Addison-Wesley editor, had the insight, provided the guidance, and did the fine-tuning. Her support and input were invaluable. The Addison-Wesley production staff, from copy editors to graphic designers, receive our sustained applause for their significant contributions. And Jane Isay, who first brought us to Addison-Wesley, must be thanked.

Special thanks go to Ruth Shiers, co-director of the Allentown–Bethlehem (Pennsylvania) Birth and Midwifery Center, for help on midwifery matters; the American College of Obstetricians and Gynecologists for providing mounds of useful information and being available as needed; Maryann Napoli, of the Center for Medical Consumers, for making available her expertise and the use of the center's library materials; Diana Korte for ongoing information and source material; and Lori Andrews for her knowledgeable insight and review of the surrogacy section.

People's Medical Society staff members also contributed their usual service beyond the call of duty. Michael Donio once again coordinated the research, made the calls, and "looked it up." Linda Swank entered much of the appendix material.

Gayle Ebert typed and mailed hundreds of letters and inquiries.

No People's Medical Society book is complete without Gail Ross, our literary agent. This is our tenth book together, with many more to come. We could not do it without her—nor would we want to!

Introduction

Modern Medicine and Pregnancy/ Childbirth: An Issue of Control

For centuries, women in labor were attended by female relatives or neighbors whose varied experience of childbirth came from having witnessed (and helped at) numerous births. Such women came to be known as midwives, from Old English roots meaning "with woman." Indeed, until the thirteenth century, women handled nearly all medical care. Historians have noted that women of that day were the doctors and anatomists, the abortionists and nurses, the counselors and the pharmacists—all without degree, but all with an unwritten license from their respective communities. But with the growth of university medical schools in Europe in the thirteenth century, medical and obstetrical skills became the sole province of male doctors.

To many historians and feminists, such as Barbara Ehrenreich and Deirdre English, the issue became one of "control: male upper-class healing under the auspices of the Church was acceptable, female healing as part of a peasant subculture was not."

And whether the control issue was intended or merely a matter of circumstance, the fact is that by the nineteenth century male doctors had captured childbirth and pronounced it inexorably a part of their domain—with the crowning blow to midwifery occurring with the advent of forceps, officially designated as a surgical instrument, which only physicians (thus effectively excluding women) were allowed to use.

Although the curtailment of midwifery started later in the United States than in Europe, ultimately the outcome was worse. As state after state banned the practice of midwifery—at a time when European midwifery was being upgraded through education and training—the medical profession came to enjoy a monopoly on childbirth care.

Along with pushing the midwife out of her role as primary caretaker of women in labor, the medical profession is responsible for shifting the setting from the home—the site of the midwife-attended birth—to the hospital. Childbirth became a pathology rather than a natural event, and doctors acquired more and more equipment with which to "treat" the "problems" associated with childbirth. Eventually, there was too much equipment to move around from house to house, so "naturally" the woman had to go to the hospital, where about 97 percent of women today give birth.

Thus occurred what many medical historians have called the "medicalization" of pregnancy/childbirth: childbirth closely controlled by physicians and hospital staff, a situation that is especially prevalent in the United States and Britain, where the physician's view of labor and delivery has moved birth from being merely a physiological process to a pathological event. Today, most American physicians advocate hospital births, directed solely by members of their profession, to the almost total exclusion of certified nurse-midwives and nonhospital delivery settings. And while this view flies in the face of evidence from countries such as the Netherlands (where 35 percent of children are born at home, mostly attended by midwives) and many other European countries where infant mortality and cesarean-section rates are far lower than ours, organized physicians' groups still maintain the "hospital as the only safe setting" mind-set. In other words, a realistic review of factual data, epidemiological evidence, and major studies on the subject suggests that physician-centered, hospital-based childbirth is only one option in a field where many other safe and appropriate options exist.

While interventionist (some would say intrusive) technology was originally developed to treat any unanticipated complications during labor or delivery, ultimately the technology developed for high-risk birth situations has come to be used for healthy, normal pregnancies.

In the meantime, something vital and valuable has been lost: the woman.

In "medicalizing" or "pathologizing" pregnancy, the medical profession has taken control of the woman's experience. In such a milieu, the doctor *delivers* a baby, instead of the woman *giving* birth. The 1950s and 1960s saw the culmination of the belief that birth should be scientifically controlled with the use of labor-induction drugs, painkillers, anesthesia, electronic monitoring, and surgical intervention (cesarean section). And with the "acceptance" of this belief, gone were all but a few midwives and home births.

Because of murmurings of dissent that began in the 1970s along with a surge in interest in so-called natural childbirth, today's obstetric practice has responded with attempts to embrace the woman's physical and emotional needs and reinstate her as an active participant in her own pregnancy and childbirth. In reclaiming lost territory, women are asserting their right to choose birth methods and determine who will be present at the birth and what technologies will be used. In the best of circumstances, what has evolved is a joint venture between the woman and her care-giver. In the worst of circumstances, pockets of old thinking still exist in many places, namely that the woman is the "child" in a parent/child relationship with her physician.

The new model, the joint venture, is the modern obstetric concept of family-centered or home*like* birth. Most doctors remain unwilling to put birthing back in the home because they want the latest technology available at a moment's notice—which means down the hall, in the hospital. Consequently, marketing-conscious hospitals now offer home*like* environments as part of the family-centered childbirth experience. There is also an upsurge in the number of certified nurse-midwives offering their services in hospitals, in free-standing midwifery centers, and, once again, in homes.

Today, you have a variety of options available, from birth

attendants to birth settings, but be aware that not every practitioner and not every hospital takes a family-centered approach. Ironically, an ever-increasing reliance on obstetrical technology—reflected in the rate of unnecessary cesarean sections—has paralleled family-centered changes.

In their book *A Good Birth, A Safe Birth* (New York: Bantam Books, 1990), childbirth educators Diana Korte and Roberta Scaer talk about some of the undercurrents in modern obstetrics: doctors' fear of malpractice suits, which too often translates into too many interventions; the readiness of insurance companies to pay for high-tech procedures (and thus reinforce doctors' urge to intervene); doctors' incomes (average net income, before taxes, for obstetricians and gynecologists in 1989: approximately $194,000) and their desire to maintain a certain level of compensation; and a sort of safety-in-numbers mentality, the peer pressure on all doctors to practice alike and not to disturb the status quo.

Whatever personal preferences you may have, whether concerning your prenatal diet, the presence of a coach (perhaps other than the baby's father) during labor and delivery, or birth position—you will have to shop around for the maternity care *you* want.

Garner all the information you can so that you can retain your birthright: a pregnancy and childbirth of your choosing.

And remember: TAKE THIS BOOK TO THE OBSTETRICIAN WITH YOU!

CHAPTER ONE

Before You Go: Prepregnancy Planning and Genetic Testing

Prepregnancy planning is a relatively new concept that presupposes that a woman and/or a couple can do much even months *before* becoming pregnant to minimize, or at least prepare for, risk during pregnancy. Some practitioners extend the time frame for prepregnancy planning to include the first few weeks of the pregnancy because of the delay in confirming pregnancy and/or the wait to get in to see a practitioner for prenatal care. Planning ahead is especially important if either the woman or her partner is at high risk of passing on inherited disorders. Clearly, pregnancy is not the optimum time to discuss such risks and any available options.

For many reasons, you may want to have a medical checkup before you become pregnant. Generally, such a checkup (or preconception testing, as it's sometimes called) includes a genetic screening and an assessment of whether you fall into any high-risk category. The usual components of the visit are medical and family history taking, a complete physical examination, and laboratory tests. Many books and experts will tell you that the obstetrician-gynecologist is the best practitioner to perform this, although it's not uncommon or necessarily undesirable for a family practitioner, internist, or midwife do so. (Be aware, however, that certain health problems may necessitate tests, screenings, and procedures out of some practitioners' domains.)

Whomever you choose, go into the consultation fully

prepared. Bring with you a list of questions, concerns, and issues you want to cover, so that the visit is more than merely expensive conversation and gets right to the point: planning for the healthiest, most satisfying pregnancy for all concerned—including your baby.

The American College of Obstetricians and Gynecologists has pinpointed the factors that the prepregnancy examination should seek to recognize. The next goal is, where appropriate, to consider, treat, or control

- poor nutritional status (whether under- or overweight);
- substance abuse (including so-called recreational drugs, smoking, excessive alcohol consumption, and use of both prescription and nonprescription drugs);
- exposure to environmental hazards;
- participation in physically demanding or hazardous activities or occupations;
- psychosocial stress;
- age;
- a large number of previous children or pregnancies;
- short intervals between earlier pregnancies;
- a history of miscarriages or stillbirths;
- a history of premature or low-birth-weight babies;
- any risk of having a child with birth defects, mental retardation, or a genetic disorder;
- susceptibility to German measles (rubella) or other infectious diseases; or
- a history of current infection with sexually transmitted diseases, streptococcal organisms, or toxoplasmosis (a disease transmitted from animals, especially cats, to humans, which during pregnancy can cause birth defects or fetal death).

Getting the Most from Your Preconception Exam

To get the most out of this consultation, have ready your personal medical history and your family history. Be sure to include your partner's family history as well, because any genetic disorders on his side may be passed on to your offspring. Using the above list as a guide, talk about the following:

- Any preexisting medical conditions, especially of a chronic nature, you have—for example, diabetes; epilepsy; high blood pressure; asthma; infections; neurological, blood, or lung disorders; or chronic inflammatory bowel disease, just to name a few of the many medical problems that can affect conception and/or pregnancy. Target your discussions on finding out *what you can do to improve your health before becoming pregnant.*

- Any medications you're taking, either prescription or nonprescription. Find out *what regimen you must/should change* for the sake of a healthy pregnancy and baby. The well-documented consequences of thalidomide use in the 1960s are a sharp, tragic reminder of the dangers of drug use during pregnancy. *Teratogens* are toxins that can cross the placenta and damage a developing fetus, causing birth defects or even fetal death, and do most of their damage in the first three months of pregnancy. One such known teratogen, the anticonvulsant Dilantin (phenytoin), has been associated with a variety of birth defects such as cleft lip or cleft palate, and other physical and mental disturbances. But discontinuing or lowering the dosages of this particular teratogenic agent should *not* be attempted *during* pregnancy because of the possible danger of seizures to the woman and the fetus, and it certainly should not be attempted without first consulting your physician. As you can see, pregnancy planning can be crucial.

- Any prior pregnancy experiences, especially miscarriage, premature birth, ectopic pregnancy, delivery complications, fetal distress, and so on. When you are in the prepregnancy planning stages, be sure to discuss risk factors, especially for ectopic pregnancy, a pregnancy in which the fertilized egg does not complete its descent but begins to develop outside the uterus, usually in one of the fallopian tubes. (This is why the term *tubal pregnancy* is used synonymously with *ectopic pregnancy*.) Ectopic pregnancy always results in the loss of the fetus and is now one of the leading causes of maternal death in this country, says the Centers for Disease Control, so every woman should be alert to the possibility of ectopic pregnancy. Talk to your doctor about the pertinence of any risk factors to your individual case *well before becoming pregnant.* Indeed, a thorough medical history in the prepregnancy planning stage

3

should raise the red flags associated with increased risk—pelvic inflammatory disease, history of endometriosis, prior tubal surgery, history of infertility, use of IUDs for contraception, and previous ectopic pregnancy. Also talk about life-style factors, such as cigarette smoking, which is emerging in new studies as a potential risk factor (*American Journal of Public Health*, September 1989).

- Life-style factors. Smoking and alcohol are the two most common environmental hazards in pregnancy, and deserve more than a passing discussion, specifically the risks involved in even reduced consumption of either nicotine or alcohol during pregnancy. Then there's the issue of acquired immune deficiency syndrome (AIDS), and the question of whom to test. Currently, the Centers for Disease Control (CDC), the American College of Obstetricians and Gynecologists, and myriad state and local health agencies recommend counseling and testing for all women of childbearing age who are at risk for the AIDS virus. The CDC's revised guidelines recommend testing for women who have used intravenous drugs; who have engaged in prostitution; whose sexual partners are infected or at risk for infection because they are intravenous drug users, are bisexual, or are hemophiliacs; who are living in communities or were born in countries where there is a known or suspected high prevalence of human immunodeficiency virus infection among women; or who had blood transfusions before blood was routinely tested for AIDS antibodies but after infection occurred in the United States.

- Any age-related concerns you have. If you are one of increasing numbers of women who have delayed childbearing into your mid- to late thirties, or beyond, you may have specific questions and concerns related to your ability to conceive in the first place, and your ability to carry and deliver a healthy baby. Experts agree that age is one of the factors involved in a healthy pregnancy, but only one. And according to the findings of a study published in the *New England Journal of Medicine* (March 8, 1990), "advancing maternal age at first birth does not appreciably increase the risk of an adverse outcome." Nevertheless, focus your discussions on certain problems that *may* increase after age thirty to thirty-five: difficulty with conception; chance of miscarriage, stillbirth, and low-birth-weight baby; rate of birth defects; and incidence of frequent chromosomal abnormalities, such as Down syndrome (Trisomy 21), the most common cause of mental retardation in this country. (We have more to say later about the prenatal tests routinely ordered for pregnant women over age thirty-five.)

• Genetic factors that may apply to you and your partner. Is there any background of twins or multiple births in your or your partner's family history? Any unusual incidence of disease or birth defects? What are some of the disorders (and their effects) you risk transmitting to your child? You have a right to know your risk for having a child with anomalies (deviations from the normal) or a genetic disorder. Find out *whether you are a carrier for a specific disease, what screenings are available to test for this, and what choices you have before you become pregnant.* Certain ethnic groups are screened for genetic disorders that are more prevalent within their groups than in the general population: for example, beta thalassemia (also called Cooley's anemia) screening in people of Mediterranean descent; Tay-Sachs screening in people of Jewish descent (specifically Eastern European, or Ashkenazic); and sickle-cell disease screening in the African-American population.

Where to Find Genetic Counseling

To find a genetic counselor or a genetic services program, or to get more information about genetic counseling, start by contacting any or all of the following groups:

• American Board of Medical Genetics (ABMG), which certifies genetics professionals and publishes a geographical roster of board-certified members. Requirements for certification include training at sites accredited by the ABMG, documentation of genetic counseling experience, evidence of continuing education, and successful completion of a comprehensive ABMG examination. Here's where to reach this group for more information: 9650 Rockville Pike, Bethesda, Maryland 20814; telephone 1-301-571-1825.

Were You a DES Baby?

Possible Complications for
Pregnancy

From the 1940s to the early 1970s, DES (diethylstilbestrol), a synthetic form of estrogen, and other, DES-type drugs were prescribed for millions of women (particularly those with pregnancy problems including bleeding, spotting, or a history of previous miscarriages) in the belief that such drugs would help prevent miscarriage. In 1971, a link was found between the use of DES during pregnancy and a rare form of vaginal cancer, and that year the Food and Drug Administration withdrew its approval of the drug for use as a pregnancy medication. Fortunately, the cancer risk is small—estimated at one in one thousand to one in ten thousand, to age thirty-two, the oldest known cancer case—according to DES Action, a non-profit consumer group providing information to the public and to health professionals about all aspects of DES exposure.

But DES daughters—that is, those exposed to DES before birth—are at higher-than-normal risk for a range of difficulties with conception and childbearing. The reports are mixed, but some studies indicate that DES-exposed women are more likely to be infertile than nonexposed women, for reasons that remain unclear. Overall, says DES Action, most DES daughters (about 82 percent) will be able to have a baby, but for many, a successful preg-

nancy may result only after serious problems or pregnancy losses.

What are the risks? And what precautions can be taken?

• Ectopic (tubal) pregnancy: Three to five times more frequent in DES daughters. Key here is to confirm as soon as possible that the pregnancy is inside and not outside the uterus, such as in a fallopian tube. Early diagnosis—usually through ultrasonography (see p. 111)—is critical, as is prompt treatment, because an ectopic pregnancy can become life-threatening.

• Early miscarriage: Evidence here is conflicting, but DES Action's position is that DES daughters seem to have more first-trimester miscarriages than other women.

• Late (second-trimester) miscarriage: About twice as frequent in DES daughters.

• Premature delivery: About twice as frequent in DES daughters.

Although often an early miscarriage is difficult to prevent, the risk of late miscarriage or early delivery can be reduced. Pat Cody, DES Action program director, says:

> Women whose mothers took the hormone DES while pregnant with them have a 1 in 2 risk for reproductive problems. If you are a DES daughter, you are considered a high-risk patient and need high-risk care from the day you know you are pregnant. If you do *not* know if you are a DES daughter, ask your

(continued)

6

mother, and/or write the medical records office of the hospital where you were born to learn if DES or diethylstilbestrol (brand name Stilbestrol) is listed on your mother's records.

High-risk care may entail everything from having more frequent examinations during pregnancy and learning to monitor for possible early contractions, or premature labor, to bed rest and labor-stopping medications.

For further information on the effects of DES exposure on daughters *and* sons, contact DES Action, 1615 Broadway, #510, Oakland, California 94612; telephone 1-415-465-4011.

- National Society of Genetic Counselors (NSGC), an organization that promotes growth and development within the profession. Unlike certification by the ABMG, which is a sign of additional training in genetics, membership in this society is open to any professional who shows an interest in the field, and it does not necessarily indicate a specialized knowledge of genetics. Nevertheless, the group may be helpful in your search for a genetic counselor and/or program because it publishes a list of genetic counseling training programs nationwide, and you can contact one near you for more information. Get in touch with the NSGC at 233 Canterbury Drive, Wallingford, Pennsylvania 19086; telephone 1-215-872-7608.

- National Center for Education in Maternal and Child Health, a government resource center that produces an up-to-date guide to genetic services centers and satellite clinics. The center also operates a clearinghouse for all sorts of publications on genetics, and if they lack materials on a topic in which you're interested, the people at the center will research it for you. The phone number for the clearinghouse is 1-202-625-8410. For more information, contact the center at 38th and R Streets, N.W., Washington, D.C. 20057; telephone 1-202-625-8400.

- National Center for Education in Maternal and Child Health and its sister organization, National Maternal and Child Health Clearinghouse, which provide education and information ser-

Genetic Counseling:

When Should You Seek It?

If you or your partner is known or suspected to have or carry a genetic disorder; if you are concerned about exposure to radiation, medications, chemicals, infection, or other substances that might pose a risk to pregnancy; if you are a woman thirty-five years of age or older; or if you have a child or other family member with mental retardation or delayed development of unknown cause, you may want to seek the services of a genetic counselor. Genetic counseling should be sought by anyone who may be at a higher risk of having a child with a birth defect or inherited disorder. At some point during the prepregnancy planning, your practitioner may recommend genetic counseling—but if not and if you believe you have just cause to be concerned, press the issue, especially if you feel your fears and concerns are being brushed off.

The goal of genetic counseling is to provide an accurate diagnosis of a known or suspected hereditary disorder, and to help people and their families manage the problems it brings about in a way that's best for them and their families. Look to the genetic counselor to answer these questions:

- Do I, my child, or another relative have a genetic disease?
- What does being a carrier mean?
- Is any member of my family a carrier of a genetic disease?
- What are the chances that my future children or other members of my family will have a particular genetic problem?
- What can be expected in the future for me or for a family member with a genetic disorder?
- Where can good treatment and care for this disorder be obtained?

What genetic counseling does not or should not do is dictate solutions. Certainties are not easy to come by. As the article "Genetic Counseling: Using the Information Wisely," in *Hospital Practice* (June 15, 1988), explains,

> [For] all the high-tech diagnostic methods we increasingly rely on, we are not really dealing with technology but with its impact on human beings. The breakthroughs in genetic diagnosis are providing us with far more information than we could have dreamed of 40 or even 30 years ago, but the problem of how to use that information wisely remains—as it always has been—difficult and elusive.

Not only are there ethical dilemmas created by the explosion of medical genetics technology and information—do you *really* want to know and what are you going to *do* with that information in hand?— but, at the same time, genetic coun-

(continued)

8

seling offers no guarantees. Having no family history of genetic defects does not guarantee that you will have a healthy infant, as the results of a study of 69,277 live-born and stillborn infants reported in the *New England Journal of Medicine* (January 5, 1989) illustrate. Of these infants, 48 were found to have serious genetic malformations even though the families of 44 percent of them had no prior history of genetic defects. And 11 malformations were caused by unexpected, new genetic abnormalities, or spontaneous mutations.

vices in maternal and child health. One of the thousands of titles available (usually free of charge) through the clearinghouse is *Comprehensive Clinical Genetic Services Centers*, a national directory of names, addresses, and contact persons of clinical genetic services centers throughout the United States that provide comprehensive diagnostic services, medical management, counseling, and follow-up care. Contact National Maternal and Child Health Clearinghouse at 38th and R Streets, N.W., Washington, D.C. 20057; telephone 1-202-625-8410.

- March of Dimes Birth Defects Foundation. Contact their national headquarters at 1275 Mamaroneck Avenue, White Plains, New York 10605; telephone 1-914-428-7100. You may also want to contact a local chapter.

You are most likely to find practicing genetic counselors at university medical centers (usually in the obstetric or pediatric department), although they also practice in private hospital settings, state or federal departments of health, private ob-gyn (obstetric-gynecology) or pediatric practices, and health maintenance organizations or other prepaid health plans. Information and technology in medical genetics is advancing so rapidly, and the evaluation entails such exact and careful interpretation of sophisticated laboratory tests, that you should consider whether anything but a specialized setting is the one for you.

Some states require that hospitals and public clinics screen for the more common genetic disorders, and there's a good chance that such screenings are done free of charge or on a sliding-scale fee. Check with your state's office of maternal and child health (the exact title of the office varies from state to state but generally operates within the department of health) for the screenings available to the public.

Throughout any and all counseling sessions you undergo, make sure you get precise information on problems that may arise from either the occurrence, or the risk of occurrence, of a genetic disorder. What are the medical facts? Diagnosis and prognosis? How serious is the disorder? What is the risk of occurrence? What choices are available for avoiding either the occurrence or recurrence? Strict birth control measures if the genetic disorder is serious and you are at high risk? Artificial insemination with donor? Adoption? What choices are available for prevention of the disorder? And—once you are pregnant—is there a prenatal test for the particular genetic disorder, one that will determine if your unborn child is affected?

Contraception and Prepregnancy Planning

You may find it surprising that matters of birth control are part of prepregnancy planning, but:

- If you have been using birth control pills, it is recommended that you switch to barrier methods for at least a month and probably for three months. This precaution helps ensure that you do not continue to take birth control pills during early pregnancy, an issue of great concern because of some possible adverse effects. This way, too, you will give your body time to reestablish its natural cycling pattern, and help improve the accuracy of the date of conception.

- If you are using an intrauterine device (IUD), experts recommend that you have it removed a month or two ahead of trying to conceive and substitute a barrier method of conception. The problem is that if you conceive while using an IUD, and if the device remains in place throughout the pregnancy, you are at greater risk of miscarriage, infection, and premature birth.

For these and many other related reasons, be sure to talk about birth control in your prepregnancy visit.

The Dangers Your Work Environment May Pose

An important part of assessing and avoiding risks during this prepregnancy planning stage is evaluating your exposure to toxic substances and other hazards on the job—some may be serious enough to warrant major changes in order to minimize the risks. But before you pose this matter to your physician or your employer, you will want to determine the greatest sources of reproductive risk *to you*. Medical writer Norra Tannenhaus, in her book *Preconceptions: What You Can Do Before Pregnancy to Help You Have a Healthy Baby* (Chicago: Contemporary Books, 1988), says the following are the greatest occupational risks:

- Chemicals and gases
- Radiation
- Vibration and loud noises
- Awkward or uncomfortable posture
- Exposure to infectious diseases
- Long hours or hard physical labor
- Emotional stress

These may affect reproductive capability, she says, in any of three ways: "They may diminish the worker's fertility. They may cause birth defects in the offspring of women who performed such jobs while pregnant. They may cause miscarriage."

Although surely you will want to discuss these potential risks with your practitioner, especially during preconceptional assessment, don't be surprised if she is unable to offer constructive advice or if her sole warning is "Remove yourself from this environment" or "Talk to your employer." Easier said than done, especially if you *must* work or if your employer is ignorant of on-the-job hazards—many do not know more than you do—or uncaring.

In any case, do not automatically trust your employer to safeguard your reproductive health. Find out for yourself what your workplace risks are. Call your state departments of environmental protection and of health. Ask about every possible hazard, from secondhand cigarette smoke to radiation, toxic chemicals, and heavy metals and solvents. Ask what nonsmoking laws your state or community has; for example, does your state/county/city mandate nonsmoking work areas and, if so, under what circumstances?

Find out whether your state has its own right-to-know law, whereby employers are required to inform workers of any risks associated with certain products with which they may be working and to provide training in protective procedures. Along with OSHA—the Occupational Safety and Health Administration in the U.S. Department of Labor—another government agency devoted to worker safety is the National Institute for Occupational Safety and Health (NIOSH). It oper-

(continued)

11

ates a toll-free telephone number for information on occupational hazards: 1-800-356-4674. Or you can write to the National Institute for Occupational Safety and Health, Department of Health and Human Resources, 4676 Columbia Parkway, Cincinnati, Ohio 45226.

Finally, throughout this prepregnancy planning stage and even after you are pregnant, be on the lookout for any sign that your practitioner considers pregnancy an illness. It is not. Pregnancy is a *healthy* state, but health in pregnancy has a lot to do with your general health before the pregnancy. Clearly, the first pregnancy visit is too late to prepare for pregnancy, and every woman can benefit from early *and* continuing risk assessment.

CHAPTER TWO

Infertility

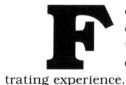or most couples, starting a family is a time of joy, excitement, and anticipation at the thought of becoming parents. But for many others, the attempt to have a child is a frustrating experience.

Infertility is defined as the inability to conceive a child after a year or more of unprotected intercourse *or* the inability to carry a pregnancy to a live birth. (Often confused with infertility, sterility is usually defined as a permanent, nontreatable, irreversible condition that prevents conception.) Over the past few decades, it has been suggested that the incidence of infertility in the United States has nearly tripled, and that now one in six American couples is infertile. Experts generally agree on two important trends to explain this phenomenon: the significant rise in sexually transmitted diseases, which can cause fertility problems, and the increasing numbers of women who are delaying childbirth until their thirties and beyond, a time when a woman's fertility begins to decline from her late twenties. Furthermore, the older a woman is, the more likely she is to have had some kind of abdominal surgery, such as an appendectomy, which may have left scarring around the reproductive organs. Tied in with the age factor is another important cause of infertility: endometriosis, a disease in which endometrial tissue, normally found in the uterus, grows outside the uterus. Women with endometriosis are only half as likely to get pregnant as women in the general population.

13

It is important to emphasize that infertility is not just a "woman's problem." Indeed, almost half of the cases of infertility are due to a male factor such as genital disease (infections and the like), an undescended testicle, blockage anywhere along the sperm route, poor sperm count or defective sperm, or hormonal disorders. In approximately 30 percent of infertile couples, both the man and the woman will be diagnosed as having fertility problems, and in 10 percent of the cases no known cause can be found. So infertility is best described as a concern for the *couple*, a perspective that is especially critical when it comes to making decisions on which tests and procedures to undergo. It is obviously foolhardy for the woman to undertake a complicated and expensive regimen—drugs, office visits, and numerous tests and treatments—when her partner has not been tested.

Treatment Options

Although not all infertile couples seek treatment, more than one million people do each year. They consult physicians for infertility evaluation and treatment, and altogether spend more than $1 billion a year to combat the problem, according to a 1988 report by the U.S. Office of Technology Assessment (OTA) (*New York Times*, May 18, 1988). Unfortunately, too often the diagnosis (or mere suspicion) of infertility starts the unwary couple on an emotionally devastating journey through a bewildering array of medical tests and procedures and often mind-boggling amounts of money. Calculating how much couples spend for infertility diagnoses and treatments, the OTA report says the figures range from a few hundred dollars to as high as $22,000, which may or may not be covered by insurance, depending on the company's plan. Yet only half of these people end up conceiving a child, and not all pregnancies result in live births.

It's hard to get in-depth information about many of today's procedures to combat infertility. Before you engage in a blind-man's buff among various tests, treatments, and practitioners, the first thing you need to know is what's available and how successful these options are. A number of medical advances,

Common Causes of Infertility

Female Factors. One of the most common causes of infertility is blockage of the fallopian tubes or other structural problems that prevent the egg and sperm from uniting. Endometriosis—a gynecological disease wherein tissue normally found in the uterus grows in other areas—is one of the many possible causes of tubal blockage. Pelvic inflammatory disease, a condition resulting from bacterial forms of sexually transmitted diseases, is another.

An equally common cause of fertility problems is ovulatory failure (failure to release an egg cell), along with other hormonal dysfunctions. The consensus among experts is that some of the greatest strides in the treatment of infertility have been made in this area, namely the development and increased effectiveness of so-called fertility drugs, which help regulate reproductive hormones.

Male Factors. A low sperm count is the most common infertility problem involving sperm production. Aside from defects in the hormonal path that ends, ultimately, with the testes, a low sperm count can be traced to a condition called a varicocele, a varicose or swollen vein in the spermatic cord. Low sperm counts may also be associated with an inguinal (groin) hernia.

Other causes include sperm that are insufficiently motile (they don't move about the way they should); sexual performance problems; blocked sperm ducts; and trauma to the scrotum and testes, which can cause scar tissue to form. Certain viral infections, including mumps, can also result in scar formation and shrinkage of the testes.

The male usually is tested first, or should be, because a semen analysis (or semenalysis) is the least stressful and most informative fertility test—actually a series of tests carried out on one sample to determine sperm levels and motility ability.

including microsurgery and more efficacious and complex pharmaceuticals, have made it possible for infertile couples to start families. Most of these so-called assisted reproductions are the result of now standard procedures.

The relatively easiest and most successful alternative to

How Do You Know If You Have a Problem?

Experts say that most couples achieve pregnancy, although it may take as long as a year or more. In a large population, 80 percent of women having regular intercourse will become pregnant within a year of trying, with an additional 5 percent pregnant by the second year. But the general consensus is that women over the age of thirty should not wait that long—one to two years—before seeking professional help. For women over thirty-five, six months is the recommended interval. Linda P. Salzer, in her book *Infertility: How Couples Can Cope* (Boston: G. K. Hall, 1986), offers some practical advice: seek help "either after one year of unsuccessful effort or at the point when anxiety is adversely affecting you or your relationship with your spouse."

natural conception is artificial insemination. Artificial insemination by husband (AIH) is the placement of the husband's semen into the wife's reproductive tract for purposes of conception, a technique generally used when the man produces a low volume of sperm. Another variation, artificial insemination by donor (AID), is often resorted to when the husband is infertile (has little or no sperm); it consists of placing donor semen into a woman's reproductive tract for purposes of conception. However, beware—not all donors are screened as carefully as perhaps *you* would want. A 1988 OTA report found that although artificial insemination is the most widely used of what it calls the "new reproductive technologies," only 44 percent of surveyed doctors test donors for AIDS, fewer than 30 percent test for syphilis and other sexually transmitted diseases, and only 48 percent screen donors for genetic disorders (*News & Comment*, August 1988).

Other traditional options available include microsurgery to repair anatomical damage and the use of fertility drugs to enhance ovulation and sperm function.

Experts estimate that these three methods are successful or effective for approximately 70 to 85 percent of all infertile couples (Geoffrey Sher, M.D., Virginia A. Marriage, and Jean Stoess, *From Fertility to In Vitro Fertilization* [New York: McGraw-Hill, 1988]).

────── ## *The High Technology of Parenting*

In vitro fertilization (IVF), a procedure used by couples for whom conventional therapies don't work, not only has received a good deal of media exposure but at the same time has left a lot of questions unanswered. IVF, recommended only after all other conventional infertility therapies have failed, is a relatively expensive endeavor—anywhere from $5,000 to $8,000 per procedure or attempt, depending on the individual program. Even faced with these astounding numbers, many couples, driven perhaps by desperation and failed attempts to achieve pregnancy, invest plenty of time, money, and emotion, no questions asked.

In vitro fertilization literally means "fertilization in glass," and was traditionally known as in vitro fertilization *and* embryo transfer. But the procedure more commonly goes by its shortened name. In vitro fertilization first made headlines in 1978 with the birth of Louise Brown, dubbed the world's first "test-tube baby," but it has come a long way since then. From the first American clinic—the Eastern Virginia Medical School at Norfolk—the number of IVF clinics in the United States has grown to around two hundred. In 1988, more than fourteen thousand procedures were performed in these clinics.

Originally developed for women with tubal infertility—that is, blocked or absent fallopian tubes—IVF is now recognized as a technique that can be effectively utilized for the treatment of infertility due to a variety of causes, including endometriosis, cervical problems, or low sperm count. As a review of the history of this technology in the May 1988 *Female Patient* concluded, however, the fact remains that "in many respects, IVF is a last-resort treatment option for patients who have failed to conceive with conventional therapies." Even if you have emotional and financial reserves beyond that of the average couple, the procedure is medically complicated, and success among the various programs nationwide varies.

17

The basic idea behind IVF is straightforward: retrieve the egg from the ovary just prior to ovulation, fertilize it in vitro—that is, bring the sperm and egg together outside the woman's body—and return the fertilized egg to the uterus. Following the transfer (admittedly the most difficult step in the process), the woman is required to remain in bed for a few days, and in many cases follow-up diagnostic procedures are done. Some couples undergo only one such treatment cycle, whereas others require two or more cycles of treatment to achieve a pregnancy.

Where Should You Seek Help? Whom Should You Consult? And How Do You Know When You Should See a Specialist?

Once you have determined that professional help is needed, where do you go? While it is true that reproductive endocrinology and fertility research have come a long way toward solving the puzzle of infertility and turning the hope of having a baby into a reality, the path to this outcome is strewn with practitioners of all sorts vying for your medical dollars.

The logical starting place is your current family physician or obstetrician-gynecologist. Bear in mind, however, that the dealings you have with the practitioner treating you for infertility will probably be very different from other doctor–consumer relationships you have had. Why? For starters, tests and treatments for infertility involve a long-term relationship with the practitioner, way beyond an office visit or two. More to the point, the issue is so emotionally charged and the stakes so high that the relationship is rife with intense hope and apprehension—on everyone's part. These are ample reasons to find a practitioner who will view you as a partner in health care and to assert your rights as a consumer.

Here are your options:

- *General or Family Practitioner, Internal Medicine Specialist (also called an Internist).* These primary care physicians can test for and solve a number of common fertility problems. Their usual starting place is a thorough medical history, physical examination, and routine lab work to determine what, if anything, in your history, environment, or medications may have had or is having an effect on your fertility. These physicians usually can do some of the initial routine tests most infertile couples go through: a semen analysis and the charting of the woman's basal body temperature (the body's lowest temperature) to discover whether she ovulates and when. Often the problem is remedied by something as relatively simple as timing intercourse to coincide with ovulation. Why waste a lot of time and money and undergo a battery of extensive fertility tests unless you absolutely need to? By the same token, however, you do not want to wait around for a practitioner to help you and run albeit routine, nevertheless useless tests only to discover that the problem is well beyond his areas of expertise.

- *Obstetrician-Gynecologist.* An ob-gyn may be a logical starting place, but bear in mind that not every ob-gyn is adequately trained or educated in infertility diagnosis and treatment. Aside from the routine pelvic exam, an ob-gyn can perform such fertility diagnostic tests as urine and/or blood tests to measure levels of various hormones; the postcoital test (examination of the woman's vaginal and cervical mucus shortly after intercourse to determine whether it and the sperm are compatible); a hysterosalpingogram (X-ray picture of the uterus, fallopian tubes, and ovaries); and an endometrial biopsy (extraction of a small piece of tissue from the uterus for examination). An ob-gyn's ability to help you beyond these and other tests depends in part on his surgical skills, specifically in microsurgery. Although most do perform some surgery, they may or may not be able to perform microsurgery on fallopian tubes, which is required in about 10 percent of infertility cases, according to Mark Perloe, M.D., and Linda Gail Christie, in *Miracle Babies and Other Happy Endings for Couples with Fertility Problems* (New York: Rawson, 1986). Many, if not most, ob-gyns can perform a laparoscopy (diagnostic examination of a woman's abdominal and pelvic cavity with a telescopic instrument inserted through a small abdominal incision), and based on the findings, the physician decides if corrective or reconstructive surgery is needed. But because microsurgery is required to do the corrective work, probably a more practical move and better use of your time and energy is to engage the services of a physician who can do both. This way a second physician does not have to repeat the laparoscopy. According to most experts, an ob-gyn should be able to perform artificial insemination and treat the problem of a failure to ovulate.

- *Reproductive Endocrinology and Fertility Specialist.* Reproductive endocrinology has been a subspecialty within obstetrics and gynecology only since 1974, and at last count there were only 370 fertility specialists board-certified by the American Board of Obstetrics and Gynecology. The American Board of Medical Specialties describes this specialist as one who has been "appropriately trained and is capable of managing complex problems relating to reproductive endocrinology [hormones] and infertility." Aside from completing an approved educational program and having an unrestricted medical license, the physician who wishes to become board-certified must pass a written examination given by the specialty board. Usually, these physicians are affiliated with infertility centers, in vitro fertilization clinics, medical schools, or major teaching hospitals.

- *Urologist.* This physician specializes in the genital-urinary system, both male and female, and is supposed to have comprehensive skills in examination of and surgery on the reproductive system and its adjacent structures. Therefore, the urologist can perform a number of procedures necessary to diagnose female or male infertility, such as examination of the testicles; analysis of quantity, quality, motility, and shape of sperm; diagnosis of endocrine, or hormonal, problems; and so on. Plus the urologist can perform a testicular biopsy, surgery for repair of a varicose vein of the spermatic cord (after infection, the second most common known cause of a low sperm count), and reversal of vasectomy.

—— Checking Credentials

You should be aware that a licensed physician may practice in any specialty and call herself a specialist in a particular field, whether or not the physician is actually board-certified in that

Fertility Tests for Women

• *Basal Body Temperature Record.* This is the tracking and recording of the body's lowest temperature in the course of a day. Because this temperature is reached during sleep, the woman takes her temperature when she wakes up in the morning—before arising, before any activity. Although far from perfect, this record can be a good indicator of ovulation, because at ovulation a woman's temperature typically dips slightly (or even remains steady) before rising a day or two after ovulation. The point of keeping a record is that three or so months of tracking should indicate the day-to-day hormone fluctuations from menstruation to ovulation, and back again.

• *Blood Tests.* These measure the hormone levels in the blood at various times during the menstrual cycle.

• *Postcoital Test.* Samples of mucus from the woman's cervix are removed after intercourse to determine if the sperm are healthy and motile, or even present at all. If they were healthy and motile during semen analysis but sluggish on the postcoital test, then there may be sperm-killing antibodies in the woman's cervical mucus.

• *Antibody Test.* This is to determine whether there are antibodies in the woman's cervical mucus that kill sperm.

• *Endometrial Biopsy.* Right before a woman is about to start her pe-riod, a few cells are scraped from the uterine lining (endometrium). Microscopic examination and analysis of the endometrium will indicate the effect of progesterone, if any, on the endometrium and whether ovulation has occurred.

• *Hysterosalpingogram.* Unlike the previously mentioned diagnostic studies, hysterosalpingogram, hysteroscopy, and laparoscopy are more complex. A hysterosalpingogram is an X-ray study of the uterus and fallopian tubes, done in order to test for structural abnormalities such as blocked tubes. This usually can be performed in the office or may be done in an outpatient setting.

• *Hysteroscopy.* This involves the visual examination of the uterus with an endoscope (a thin, flexible tube with fiber-optic viewing capabilities) inserted through the vagina and the cervix. Again, the purpose is to test for structural problems that may be preventing conception from taking place. According to Joe Noumoff, M.D., of the Hospital of the University of Pennsylvania, the preferred location for performing this procedure is the hospital operating room. This is not to say, of course, that there aren't some doctors with in-office "scopes" doing the procedure there.

• *Laparoscopy.* Actually a surgical procedure because it involves a small abdominal incision (and either general or local anesthesia), laparoscopy is a visual examination of
(continued)

the abdominal and pelvic organs via a telescopic instrument. Depending on what is found—scar tissue around reproductive organs or other anatomical abnormalities—reconstructive surgery may be recommended. Opinion is somewhat divided over the best setting in which to perform this procedure, with some experts reporting it safely done on an outpatient basis and others saying it requires hospitalization. There are some, too, who maintain that it can be done safely under sedation and with local anesthesia in a doctor's office.

specialty. At the very least, determine that the physician is who and what she purports to be, knowledgeable and skilled in that specialty or area of expertise. A good way to begin is to find out whether or not she is board-certified—that is, has the physician spent a number of years in postgraduate training and passed a certifying examination? Also, keep in mind that while not a guarantee of competence, board certification is a minimum standard of excellence—many would say *the* minimum standard—for choosing a doctor today.

To verify the credentials of any physician claiming to hold board certification in a medical specialty, you can:

- Call or write the appropriate board:

  American Board of Obstetrics and Gynecology
  4225 Roosevelt Way, N.E., Suite 305
  Seattle, Washington 98105
  Telephone: 1-206-547-4884

  American Board of Internal Medicine
  University City Science Center
  3624 Market Street
  Philadelphia, Pennsylvania 19104
  Telephone: 1-215-243-1500

  American Board of Urology
  31700 Telegraph Road, Suite 150
  Birmingham, Michigan 48010
  Telephone: 1-313-646-9720

- See if your public library or a local hospital library has a copy of the *American Medical Directory: Directory of Physicians in the United States, Puerto Rico, Virgin Islands, Certain Pacific Islands, and U.S. Physicians Temporarily Located in Foreign Countries.* This lists every doctor: his year of license; primary/ secondary specialty; type of practice; board certification; and premedical and medical school education. Another valuable source is the *Directory of Medical Specialists*, published by Marquis Who's Who, Macmillan Directory Division.

- Contact RESOLVE, a national self-help group for infertile individuals and couples: 5 Water Street, Arlington, Massachusetts 02174; telephone 1-617-643-2424. RESOLVE has more than fifty chapters throughout the United States, and the national office can give you the address and telephone number of the one nearest you. Aside from telephone counseling, local support groups, and public education, RESOLVE also offers referral services. You may find it helpful to attend a local meeting and ask the members about their experiences with various doctors.

- Contact the American Fertility Society (AFS), which can provide you with a list of physicians in your area who are members of the organization: 2140 11th Avenue South, Suite 200, Birmingham, Alabama 35205-2800; telephone 1-205-933-8494. Membership in the American Fertility Society—with its attendant emphasis on disseminating up-to-date information on all aspects of infertility—is available to any practitioner expressing an interest in the area of reproductive medicine, but does not guarantee a standard of training, experience, or expertise. Nonetheless, the interest alone is a definite plus. (The American Fertility Society has affiliated societies, which any AFS member may join after certain criteria have been met: Society of Reproductive Endocrinologists, for AFS members who also have certificates of special competence in reproductive endocrinology from the American Board of Obstetrics and Gynecology; and Society of Reproductive Surgeons, for AFS members judged to have the special training, experience, and competence necessary for fertility surgery.)

- Contact the Society for Assisted Reproductive Technology (SART), also affiliated with the American Fertility Society: 2140 11th Avenue South, Suite 200, Birmingham, Alabama 35205-2800; telephone 1-205-933-8494. SART can provide you with a list of all IVF programs that actively perform IVF, GIFT, or related advanced reproductive technologies *and* that meet minimum standards, specifically: completion of a minimum of forty cycles per year, birth of three infants to three different mothers as a result of IVF, and submission of its data to the national registry (which publishes an annual report in *Fertility and Sterility*, the official journal of the American Fertility Society).

- Question, question, question! Call the office, clinic, center, or whatever and ask what training—besides obstetrics and gynecology—qualifies the doctor to evaluate and treat infertility.

How do you know when you should go beyond your primary care physician and see a fertility specialist?

If pregnancy does not occur within a year or so (and less for some women beyond their twenties) of unprotected intercourse, your physician should order some basic tests: blood and urine tests, semen analysis, postcoital test, and so on. (Some women's health centers do basic infertility testing, and some offer reduced fees for low-income patients or those without insurance coverage.) If these basic tests indicate a problem that is out of your physician's purview, or if infertility continues, then perhaps it is time to consult a specialist. It's also a good idea to do so if you have suffered a number of miscarriages—some experts say three or more—or if, as we said before, infertility is affecting your relationship with your partner or your own self-esteem.

If you do go on to seek the help of a specialist, make sure your medical record and any test results from consultations with previous physicians are passed on to this specialist so that you won't waste your time and money on more of the same. Also, arrange for *both* you and your partner to attend consultations. This way you both can air personal concerns, ask questions, and plan the course of your workup.

Infertility tests, surgery, and drugs are expensive, and few are without some risks. To get the most out of this specialist consultation, you must question the doctor, specifically on what she wants to do on or to you. Question the necessity *and* the cost of each and every test or procedure:

■ *What will you be looking for in the results of these tests?*

This is a key question because it requires your doctor to let you in on the process, diagnosis, and prognosis, and to justify the need for further testing.

■ *Can this test/procedure be performed in your office? In a hospital outpatient department?*

Since a test may require hospitalization, and given all the potential hazards that involves—in-hospital infections, drug mishaps, medication errors, and the like—you certainly will want to discuss this matter ahead of time.

■ *How much will this test/procedure/program cost?*

Insurance coverage for infertility tests and treatments historically has been hit-and-miss. It is critical to find out up front what *all* the costs will be.

■ *How much time will it take—how long, what time of day, and how close are the multiple visits? Will I be incapacitated? Will I miss work?*

These questions are not as selfish and trivial as they may seem. The testimonies of couple after couple attest to the strain of infertility treatment on their work and personal lives, especially because the treatment often involves intercourse and tests "on schedule." Losing work time, much-needed pay, and maybe even your job itself are all possibilities. When you have the information, discussions with your doctor and employer will help you to determine if you can afford to—or not afford to—pursue a certain medical course.

■ *Do the potential advantages of the procedure/test outweigh the procedure's/test's risks?*

Ask if any procedure or test is dangerous or can cause serious problems as a side effect. Ask about the risk of multiple birth, ectopic pregnancy, and so on. Have your doctor give you a rundown on any and all possibilities.

■ *Is this the most appropriate test?*

Tests are big money for doctors and facilities. Today, any number of tests are used to diagnose or rule out infertility. Because of this, many doctors have fallen victim to "testitis"— they use all the tests available instead of the most comprehensive one. Watch out for the doctor who wants to move you up the test ladder. Ask why he is not recommending the most comprehensive one *first*. Remember, one comprehensive test may be much cheaper than three lesser ones.

Often, infertility therapy involves potent drugs. Take the use of hormones to induce ovulation because of the difficulty of pinpointing exactly when a woman will ovulate. Pergonal (the trade name for human menopausal gonadotropin, or HMG) is a prime example of the need to ask many questions before and during treatment. Writing in her book *New Conceptions* (New York: St. Martin's Press, 1984), Lori B. Andrews, J.D., says: "Extremely careful monitoring is necessary when a woman uses gonadotropins . . . [substances] so powerful that they can overstimulate the ovary, causing it to enlarge, painfully swelling up the abdominal cavity, and sometimes causing blood pressure to fall. In severe cases the woman will need to be hospitalized." She concludes, "It is important to undergo Pergonal therapy only with a doctor who is thoroughly familiar with the drug." And more experts cite other risks: Pergonal therapy is associated with multiple birth and the development of multiple ovarian cysts.

So some of the same intense questions apply to medication therapy: "What results do you expect from the medication? How long and often must I take it? What will it cost? What are the side effects and/or adverse reactions? What are the risks?"

What Price Pregnancy?
And Who Pays What?

Along with making sure both you and your partner work together with the practitioner, discussing all recommendations before plunging ahead, and asking questions at every turn, another way to stay in control of a situation that has snowballed disastrously for many couples is to tailor the diagnostic workup and therapeutic program to your emotional needs *and* budget. And this means exploring who pays what.

You will (or should, if the practitioner is willing to work on an equal partnership basis with you—the only way to fly) find out a lot about costs of tests and procedures by asking the questions we outlined earlier. Also ask whether you must pay in advance or whether the physician will send the bills to your insurance carrier. (By the way, just about everyone we talked to said to expect to pay something up front.)

The going rate for a full diagnostic workup that includes both partners is somewhere between $1,500 and $3,000, according to the Office of Technology Assessment, and involves multiple office visits and often a day in the hospital. Of course, follow-up treatment frequently runs as high as $8,000. True, a number of couples, sometime during the evaluation phase, will achieve pregnancy without any specific treatment, but many others face mounting costs and the question of where it all will end.

Most couples depend on their health insurance to cover all or most of the expenses, but here the story is not all good. Insurance companies often refuse to pick up the tab or, at the very least, they curtail coverage for infertility claims. It is all fine and good to find out up front what the costs will be, and we heartily recommend you press your practitioner to do so (no matter how impatient he becomes with this consumerist approach), but a complicating factor is that it's difficult to predict how much procedures will cost. Therefore, it's difficult to assess what your insurance will and will not pay.

The sticking point is that insurers do not consider infertility a bona fide medical problem—it's not an illness or an injury. They also argue that in vitro fertilization and other advanced procedures "bypass rather than actually fix the problem," according to a *Wall Street Journal* report (December 5, 1989). Insurers generally cover diagnostic work, but treatment is another story. Some companies outright exclude infertility treatments, especially the newer procedures such as in vitro fertilization, because they consider the treatments experimental. Another advanced, new procedure is gamete intrafallopian transfer (GIFT), in which retrieved eggs and treated sperm are placed into the fallopian tubes, and from there fertilization and pregnancy can take place as they normally do. Even Massachusetts, a state whose insurance laws most extensively cover infertility treatments, denies coverage for GIFT, citing its experimental nature.

A 1987 survey by the Health Insurance Association of America found that only one out of four of their member companies covers in vitro under group policies, with large companies more likely to reimburse. Insurers cite the low success rate of in vitro, which in combination with high costs, they say, argues against coverage.

The *Wall Street Journal* article does report, however, that about 70 percent of other infertility procedures (hormone treatments and surgery to repair reproductive organs) are insured, but even here coverage is inconsistent.

Undoubtedly, the debate will continue, but thanks to the efforts of consumer groups, including RESOLVE, the infertility support group leading the fight to gain backing for infertility insurance, the picture is becoming less gloomy. Six states—Arkansas, Hawaii, Maryland, Massachusetts, Rhode Island, and Texas—currently require insurance companies to cover infertility treatments, including in vitro fertilization. And even in states where coverage is not expressly mandated, insurers do pay for IVF, but on a case-by-case basis.

How can you lessen your chances of being bankrupted by infertility treatments? We'll say it again: start by talking the whole matter over with your physician—what services will probably be required, what is likely to be covered, and what arrangements can be made to parcel out your share of payments. Here are some other tips:

- Assume nothing where insurance coverage is concerned. Even in states that mandate coverage, certain restrictions may apply. In Maryland, for example, the mandate excludes self-insured companies.

- Get a copy of your insurance policy and check it over carefully for limitations and exclusions. If your policy does not specifically list these, or even just to guarantee that you have all the facts straight, contact your company benefits manager or the insurer itself and determine how infertility claims are treated. And ask for a written copy of this declaration!

- Find out if your insurance plan has dollar limits or caps in place. At least one state, Arkansas, has set a lifetime cap of $15,000 on infertility treatments.

- Bear in mind that prepaid insurance plans, such as health maintenance organizations (HMOs) or preferred provider organizations, operate quite differently from traditional health insurance. According to a report in March 1989 *Changing Times*, "HMOs will cover infertility treatments in states that mandate it, but otherwise you're on your own. Specialists are few and far between at most centers and coverage may not extend beyond diagnosis." A 1988 Group Health Association of America survey of HMOs with at least three years' track record found that only 17 percent covered in vitro fertilization.

- Take advantage of the federal income tax deduction for medical expenses by clustering all infertility tests and treatments in a single year, if possible. Of course, there are certain exclusions and requirements that you first must investigate.

- Set a time *limit* on treatment. Most assuredly, this is tough, and every couple will have different benchmarks, but an endless round of tests, treatments, and bills can bankrupt both your financial *and* emotional reserves. Many infertile couples will try almost anything, no matter how costly, and too often push themselves beyond their ability to pay *and their ability to cope*. As Salzer, in *Infertility: How Couples Can Cope*, put it: "Somewhere it is said that infertility patients are second only to terminal cancer patients in their willingness to tolerate any kind of medical treatment." And too often, we might add, pay all the while.

- Seek a second opinion anytime you feel you're not making progress, or anytime your doctor is not engaging in honest, open communication or not answering your questions satisfactorily.

- Find out under what business or management arrangement the clinic or center operates. Is it for-profit? Affiliated with a medical school or research center? This information is a matter of public record and, if asked about, must be disclosed. In *Miracle Babies*, Perloe and Christie weigh the advantages of a private physician versus a large fertility clinic and conclude that (1) "Research-oriented clinics may perform unnecessary tests and procedures to meet research criteria and pay their expenses," (2) "For-profit fertility clinics tend to charge more for basic diagnostic workups and treatments than do family practitioners and obstetrician-gynecologists," and (3) "Many communities are not large enough to support fertility specialists and in vitro clinics . . . [therefore] traveling to distant medical facilities may add unnecessarily to your out-of-pocket expenses, absenteeism from work, and overall level of stress."

——— Settings Fertile for Misrepresentation

To the infertile couple desperately seeking the most appropriate, most successful medical technology to achieve pregnancy, in vitro fertilization or any of the other options can look like miraculous answers. But how can you, a consumer and probably not in a medical profession, find out whether one program or procedure is any better than the next? Question, question, question, is what we've been urging you to do all along, and the same dictum holds true here. How do you know whether a fertility clinic you have chosen can deliver?

As fertility clinics, IVF programs, and the like have sprung up nationwide, quality of treatment has become a major concern—and for good reason. During more than a decade of growth, there has been a lack of clear, unbiased information about the performance of in vitro fertilization clinics, and the field remains largely unregulated by federal and state governments.

But consumers now have their best information so far on the track record of clinics that use high-technology techniques to produce babies. The information comes from the first national survey of such clinics released in 1989, a combined effort of the House Subcommittee on Regulation, Business Opportunities, and Energy and the American Fertility Society. The survey's findings, in brief: clinics offering in vitro fertilization services to infertile couples vary widely in success rates. The congressional report also said that some of the clinics "overstate" in their advertisements their success rates of resultant births. According to a *New York Times* (March 10, 1989) article, of the 165 surveyed clinics that said they perform in vitro fertilization, the average reported success rate—measured in live births—was 11 percent for 1987 and 1988 "when using a conservative way of calculating these figures." But some clinics advertise rates up to three times higher or cite other figures that imply greater success, without making clear what the numbers mean.

A 1989 General Accounting Office report found that half of the IVF programs surveyed had less than a 14 percent success rate (defined as live birth or a second- or third-trimester pregnancy) in 1988. The highest success rate reported among the 160 IVF programs surveyed was 38 percent, and 9 percent of the programs had no successes, down substantially from a survey the year before which found that half of the nation's IVF clinics hadn't produced a live baby.

Speaking at a conference in 1987, Daniel R. Mishell, Jr., M.D., chairman of the department of obstetrics and gynecology at Women's Hospital–Los Angeles County, University of Southern California Medical Center, advised telling IVF patients the truth about rates of pregnancy. His definition of the truth? "The chances of taking a baby home per in vitro fertilization cycle are 5 to 7 percent, and the patient must be prepared to undergo at least six treatment cycles to improve her chances for success" (*Ob. Gyn. News*, March 1–14, 1987). In a letter to the editor in the *New England Journal of Medicine* (October 12, 1989), a physician and two associates researching IVF success rates write: "We conclude that the overwhelming majority of couples who will achieve pregnancy as a result of IVF do so within a relatively short period of time. Couples who do not achieve a viable pregnancy after four to six cycles should be counseled that success with this technique is unlikely and should not be encouraged to pursue IVF any further."

IVF is an expensive last resort for infertile couples. And if the procedure is unsuccessful—that is, does not result in a live birth, a baby to take home, which it very often does not— you've paid a lot of money to have your heartfelt hopes dashed.

The hedging on success rates has to do with how the clinic measures success, by what definition. Egg retrieval and fertilization of embryos are ways to measure success rates, but there are others. Some of the clinics inflating their success rates are counting *all* conceptions as successes, even if they end in miscarriage or otherwise fail, as 30 percent do. And some count as pregnancies even those cases in which blood tests show elevated hormone levels but pregnancy does not occur. Or a clinic may calculate the rate over a short interval and not over years.

Don't be misled by a program's success story. And by no means buy the services of an IVF clinic that's playing fast and loose with the facts. One of the best measures of success is the number of live births. As a group of Canadian ob-gyns writing in the *Canadian Medical Association Journal* (January 15, 1989) put it: "The take-home-baby rate in our opinion is the most meaningful statistic to couples contemplating IVF." What reasonable success rate should you look for in an IVF program? Experts say somewhere between 10 and 15 percent.

Another area of concern raised by the congressional survey is the lack of regulation. The Federal Trade Commission and other government and professional organizations provide little if any oversight of in vitro fertilization practices, which are performed in a variety of settings ranging from giant university medical complexes to single-doctor offices. So it is critical that you arm yourself with all the knowledge and facts that you can muster.

Copies of the congressional survey (*Consumer Protection Issues Involving IVF Clinics*) are in depository libraries throughout the country. To get the name of the one nearest you, contact your local library. If you wish, you may purchase a copy of the survey (stock number 552-070-06387-1) for $31 from the Government Printing Office: Superintendent of Doc-

How Do You Spell Success?

The American Fertility Society recommends that a couple ask the following questions to understand the true success story of any IVF clinic they're considering:

1. When did this program perform its first IVF procedure? First GIFT procedure?
2. How many babies have been born from this program's IVF efforts? GIFT efforts?
3. In the past two years, how many stimulation cycles have been initiated for IVF? For GIFT?
4. In the past two years, how many egg recovery procedures have been done in the IVF program? GIFT program?
5. In the past two years, how many embryo transfer procedures have been done in the IVF program?
6. In the past two years, how many pregnancies have resulted from IVF? From GIFT?
7. In the past two years, how many miscarriages have occurred from pregnancies initiated by IVF? By GIFT?
8. In the past two years, how many live births have occurred in your program from IVF? From GIFT?
9. How many ongoing pregnancies are there from IVF? From GIFT?
10. How many deliveries were twins or other multiple births?

The American Fertility Society's excellent pamphlet *Questions to Ask about an IVF/GIFT Program* explains three ways to determine a program's "take-home baby" rate:

The first two equations are based on egg recovery procedures, and the third is based on embryo transfers. For IVF or GIFT, divide live births (question 8) by egg recovery procedures (question 4); or, add live births (question 8) to ongoing pregnancies (question 9) and divide the sum by egg recovery procedures (question 4). In the latter equation, which can be applied to the most recent results of a program, you are assuming the ongoing pregnancies will result in live births. For IVF, divide live births (question 8) by embryo transfers (question 5).

uments, Congressional Sales Office, U.S. Government Printing Office, Washington, D.C. 20402; telephone 1-202-275-3030.

If you are considering using the services of a fertility clinic, what can you do to get the best care for your investment of time, money, and emotion?

- Find a clinic with a board-certified endocrinologist and/or a board-certified obstetrician-gynecologist on staff. But a clinic with a whole range of appropriate specialties on the consultative team is even better.

- Ask about the doctor's training in in vitro fertilization—when and where. Is the doctor board-certified in reproductive endocrinology? Find out how many procedures she has performed, and remember that any advanced technique takes time to learn. Experience is important.

- Find out how many doctors will be involved in your care and whether your doctor (if you wish) can participate in your care.

- Ask how long the clinic has been in business and how many clients it has. The more volume a program has, the higher the chances are that the medical experts will have treated all types of complex infertility problems.

- Ask if the program meets the American Fertility Society's minimal standards. These standards require IVF/GIFT programs to have staff trained in reproductive endocrinology, laparoscopic surgery, sonography, hormone measurement, tissue culture technique, and sperm–egg interaction. Does the program report its results to the IVF Registry? Participation is voluntary in this ongoing collection of IVF/GIFT results, published annually in the American Fertility Society's journal *Fertility and Sterility*. The minimal standard for IVF clinics recommended by the American Fertility Society and other experts is at least forty egg retrieval attempts a year and three or more live births. Remember, this is a *minimal standard*. David Hill, Ph.D., director of Los Angeles–based Century City Hospital's IVF program, for instance, maintains that a quality program will see upward of fifteen cases a month, preferably twenty.

- Don't be fooled by membership in professional societies. Membership in the American Fertility Society and its affiliated group, Society for Assisted Reproductive Technology, connotes an interest in fertility problems but indicates no special expertise, training, or skills. At this time, there are no special credentials or standards *required* for a doctor to perform any infertility treatment.

- Find out the clinic's success rate for the particular infertility problem you have. Ask the specialist, the clinic director, whomever you can think of, what the success rate is in achieving full-term pregnancies and live births. Also ask what *your* particular chances are for success, given your specific medical circumstances, age, and so on.

- Ask about waiting lists. You may have been treated through several frustrating years of infertility before coming to try IVF or some other advanced medical technology, and the fact that a program has a six-month or more waiting list will be important to know.

- Ask what happens after a procedure is canceled—where will you fall on the waiting list? Typically, infertile couples do not go through a repeat IVF procedure, one after the other, without a time lapse or "rest cycle" in between.

- Search for a clinic that has a counseling referral service or itself offers psychological counseling for infertile couples. (Find out, too, whether the sessions are included in the cost of the procedure.) In vitro fertilization and its variations are emotionally charged procedures, and far too few centers routinely provide psychological counseling. Also ask about available support groups.

- Ask about the clinic's payment schedule and whether it accepts insurance payment. Sliding-scale fees—that is, based on ability to pay—are desirable.

Finally, you should be aware that, whether overt or not, many IVF programs screen potential clients and, according to a May 1988 *Ms.* magazine special report, this practice "makes [IVF] inaccessible to most women." Quoting an expert who worked on The Reproductive Laws for the 1990s Project, which brought together a diverse group of experts in many fields, the article says, "Most in vitro clinics are highly selective, accepting only married, heterosexual women with adequate resources."

There you have it—ask a lot of questions and be prepared to walk out the door if you don't get the answers you need, or any answers at all. Remember: it's your body, it's your time, it's your money. And be sure to take advantage of groups offering information, educational materials, counseling, and other services.

Technological Spin-offs of IVF

You should be familiar with variations—some call them refinements—of in vitro fertilization that are gaining ground in the marketplace of reproductive technology.

Gamete Intrafallopian Transfer (GIFT). This variation is one we've already touched on. Similar to IVF in its use of ovulation-inducing drugs, egg retrieval, ultrasound examinations, and blood tests, GIFT is a process in which the retrieved eggs and treated sperm are placed directly in the fallopian tubes for fertilization to occur as it normally would, in vivo. GIFT is available only to women with at least one normal, unobstructed fallopian tube and one healthy ovary, but it may be appropriate for some male fertility problems and cervical mucus or sperm antibody problems. The procedure is used most often for couples with unexplained infertility and minimal endometriosis and, therefore, may result in a higher pregnancy rate due to the types of women being treated. Because a laparoscopy or a minilaparotomy (a small incision made in the abdomen above the pubic bone) must be done to place the eggs, GIFT's chief disadvantage over modern IVF is that it is invasive. Although precise data are hard to come by, estimates are that the pregnancy rates for GIFT "are the same as or slightly higher than for in vitro fertilization" (*New England Journal of Medicine*, March 31, 1988). As to the chance of giving birth, a *U.S. News & World Report* (April 3, 1989) article places this at close to 20 percent with GIFT, according to 1988 data. Its cost approaches that of IVF, and for this and other reasons GIFT should be considered a last resort after less invasive therapeutic methods have been explored.

Zygote intrafallopian transfer (called ZIFT) is a new variation of GIFT. In this process, the egg is fertilized in vitro and the embryo placed in the fallopian tube about eighteen hours later. Reports warn that the procedure is too new for its success to be measured.

Embryo Transfer. Generally speaking, embryo transfer is the procedure used to place a living embryo into a woman's uterus, but up to this point we have discussed the process as it relates to IVF and the infertile couple: her egg and his sperm. In the most current sense of the term, embryo transfer involves a third person, a woman who is a volunteer donor. In this procedure, the man's sperm are used to fertilize the egg of the volunteer donor via artificial insemination. After several days, the embryo is washed from the womb of the surrogate, and if fertilization has occurred, the embryo is transferred to the recipient's uterus for gestation. The key to the transfer process is the precise synchronization of the menstrual cycles of two women. In the present sense, embryo transfer is considered a solution for the woman who is unable to conceive but is able to carry a child to term. There are some risks to the donor, however, specifically the chance that she remains pregnant because the embryo is not washed out with the fluid, or the chance that she is left with an ectopic pregnancy should the embryo be flushed back into the fallopian tube.

Embryo Freezing. Not exactly a variation but certainly a spin-off of IVF, embryo freezing (cryopreservation) is another option for the infertile couple. It is available in some IVF programs. In *New Conceptions*, Andrews describes the process and its potential advantages:

> Hormone stimulation of a woman's ovaries during the IVF process may lead to the release of more than one egg. In most current IVF programs, if a number of eggs are removed and fertilized, all the ones that are developing are implanted in the woman. This had led to the birth of several pairs of twins. . . . With embryo freezing, the woman could bring to term some of the embryos and "save" the other embryos to be reimplanted at a later date.

This way, too, the woman does not have to repeat the process of retrieving and fertilizing eggs, because embryo freezing offers the possibility of pregnancy beyond the initial treatment cycle.

Andrews cautions that the use of frozen embryo banks "gives rise to myriad legal concerns. . . . Who is responsible for a frozen embryo if the couple die? If a couple divorce and no longer want the embryo, can it be given to another infertile couple? . . . For inheritance purposes, should a frozen embryo be considered an extra child?" Then there's the possible use of frozen embryo banks "in which embryos are produced to order by matching the sperm and ovum of 'ideal' types and then sold to parents for genetic or eugenic purposes"—a matter raised by leading medical ethicist George J. Annas, J.D., and Sherman Elias, M.D., in an article in *Clinical Obstetrics and Gynecology* (September 1989).

—— *Surrogacy: Is This an Option for You?*

Today, there are more ways to have a baby than most of us ever dreamed of. But as the technology of reproduction continues its rapid advance, not every scientific or social breakthrough is right for everyone. Surrogacy, or surrogate motherhood, exemplifies this dilemma. It is probably the most controversial and compelling of the new conceptions. Even though surrogate centers have been serving as matchmakers for surrogates and couples since the late 1970s, surrogacy remained a quiet issue; primarily infertile couples, and some lawyers and clergy, were the only ones struggling with the complexities involved. All that changed in late 1986 when the Baby M case made the headlines, and, by the time that case came to trial in 1987, worldwide attention was focused on the issue, and debates raged (and continue to) in living rooms, conference centers, courtrooms, and state legislatures nationwide.

First, what is surrogacy? Typically, the husband is fertile, but the wife is not—or is not able to carry the pregnancy to term. Another woman volunteers to become pregnant with the husband's sperm, through artificial insemination, and carry the pregnancy. (There is another, less common variation, called IVF surrogacy, in which the couple's embryo is implanted in a surrogate, who then carries the pregnancy.) After the baby is born, the man who provided the sperm is the legal father and the surrogate mother allows the father's wife to adopt the baby.

Of course, not all is smooth sailing, as the Mary Beth Whitehead, or Baby M, case illustrates. Whitehead decided to break the contract she had with William and Elizabeth Stern—in which for $10,000 she agreed to bear a child for Stern—and decided to keep the child. The rest, as the saying goes, is history: in March 1987 a New Jersey courthouse was the scene of the first American custody case involving a child born to a surrogate mother. The result of the landmark nonjury trial? The judge placed Baby M with the Sterns, terminated Whitehead's parental rights, and allowed Elizabeth Stern to adopt the baby. On appeal, the New Jersey Supreme Court put Whitehead back in the role of legal mother. The Sterns retained custody, but a lower court granted Whitehead certain visitation rights. Just as important as the details of adoptive parenthood and custody is the impact of the Baby M case on state legislatures where, after years of procrastination and foot-dragging, their thoughts finally turned to surrogacy.

Since then, a few dozen states have considered legislation on surrogacy, ranging from regulation to outright prohibition, and two states (Florida and Michigan) have made it illegal to enter into or arrange a surrogate-parent contract that pays a fee to the surrogate mother. Even in the few states that have enacted laws on surrogacy, most do not clearly specify who gets the child if the contract is disputed—a critical exclusion since the couple's major risk is that the surrogate mother will decide to keep the baby after birth. In spite of this and the media attention surrounding the Whitehead case, Lori B. Andrews, J.D., in *Between Strangers: Surrogate Mothers, Expectant Fathers, and Brave New Babies* (New York: Harper & Row, 1989), reminds us that in reality only 1 percent of surrogate mothers change their minds about relinquishing the child.

Nevertheless, surrogacy is a complex issue, and like all

contractual arrangements—much less one as explosive and controversial as this—it calls for much soul-searching and even legal advice. And, in fact, it's not far wrong or too facetious to suggest that you take this particular reproductive matter to the lawyer (and not the obstetrician) with you.

Given the complex legal and moral issues involved in surrogacy, seemingly endless questions have to be explored and answered, if possible, not the least of which is the question of whether this is for you. If you cannot carry a pregnancy—you have no uterus, you have no ovaries, you don't respond to other therapies, you carry a genetic disease, or you have health problems that preclude pregnancy—then surrogacy is a viable alternative. But this just scratches the surface. Other questions explore your inner motivations and possible responses to an arrangement that someone has described as a "Pandora's box." Do you choose someone you know or someone previously unknown to you? How emotionally troublesome will the relationship between the surrogate mother and your husband be? How will you perceive the relationship? What role, if any, will jealousy play? With contact between the child and the surrogate mother a possibility in the future, how will you react to their relationship, their biological bond? What if the surrogate mother wants visitation privileges? How will you handle the reaction of family and friends to the surrogate arrangement? What will you tell the child about the circumstances? What if the child is born with a disability?

Of course, you will never know for certain all the answers until the situation moves from the hypothetical to the real, and then you must consider the practical and legal realms of surrogacy. Just remember, above all, to examine these issues thoroughly beforehand. Carefully consider whether it is right for you and, if so, when, where, and how.

Private arrangements for a surrogate can be made, but about twenty-four surrogate programs currently exist (with more reputedly on the way) for the purpose of facilitating such arrangements. Although costs vary from program to program, expect the price tag to be considerable. (Costs can run $20,000 and higher.) And expect to ask a lot of questions. In *Infertility: How Couples Cope*, Salzer recommends a few:

■ *How are surrogates screened, medically and psychologically?* (And—we might add—do the surrogate and the couple have veto power over one another?)

The psychological screening primarily serves to ensure that the surrogate understands the agreement and will be willing to give up the child after birth, and that the arrangement will not harm her in any way.

■ *What are the legal responsibilities and rights of all involved?*

A particular sticking point here has been whether the biological father should have control over the surrogate mother's medical treatment during the pregnancy. Many contracts have stipulated, for example, that the surrogate mother agree to amniocentesis and, if the test reveals a genetic defect, that she agree to an abortion. Some contracts even prohibit the surrogate from drinking alcohol, smoking, and taking drugs while she's pregnant. In a spring 1988 *Law, Medicine & Health Care* article, Andrews points out, however, that "most [legislative] bills regulating surrogacy that have been proposed in recent years specifically state that the surrogate shall have control over medical decisions during the pregnancy." Other contentious issues are what rights the husband has if the surrogate refuses to relinquish the child and whether the surrogate should have a grace period, similar to adoption, after the birth to assert her parental rights.

■ *What contact is there between the couple and the surrogate?*

You should be aware that some surrogacy centers require complete confidentiality, in which neither the surrogate mother nor the couple knows each other's identity. Most programs approach the matter of contact by arranging face-to-face visits, going so far in some cases as to encourage the surrogate mother and the couple to form a close relationship.

■■ *Is psychological counseling provided?*

Without a doubt, a surrogate arrangement can be emotionally taxing to all parties involved, no matter how "prepared" they feel. Realizing this, some centers require that the surrogate mother and the couple participate in counseling sessions. Counseling may also serve to establish what each party wants out of the relationship and carefully match the surrogate with the couple.

There's no doubt about it: reproductive choices are tough choices, and this is true in spades with surrogacy. So arm yourself with knowledge and a healthy, consumerist skepticism, and take advantage of all the resources you can find. If surrogacy is an arrangement you are seeking, the very first information you need is whether your state has a law specifically dealing with surrogacy. (Remember, few states do.) Call the family law section of your state's bar association to find out. If there is such a law, what restrictions apply? (Most states have no specific surrogacy laws. Those that do tend to prohibit court enforcement of paid surrogacy contracts, rather than ban the arrangement itself.) In the absence of a specific law, find out what laws or precedents govern such arrangements.

CHAPTER THREE

Choosing a Birth Practitioner

The commonly held wisdom in the field of obstetrics is that 90 percent of all pregnant women are capable of delivering normally without any help or interference, and some experts even say this is a conservative figure—that somewhere between 93 and 96 percent is more realistic.

Even with the medical intervention that occurs in the majority of births in this country—namely, that 97 percent of births take place in hospitals and usually with doctors as birth practitioners—most women go through pregnancy and delivery with few or no complications.

Doctors do make mistakes, however. Improper birth-related treatment has consistently placed high on the list of the top ten malpractice claims compiled annually by St. Paul Fire and Marine Insurance Company, the largest private malpractice insurer in the country. In 1988, improper birth-related treatment was the second most frequent malpractice allegation, behind "postsurgery complications" at number one and ahead of "failure to diagnose cancer," the third most frequent allegation. For that year, the company tallied the average cost (defense expenses, plus any trial award or settlement) per birth-related malpractice claim at $129,123. Failure to diagnose pregnancy problems, a category of malpractice claims that in previous years appeared in the top ten, didn't make the list in 1988; nevertheless, plenty of errors continue to be committed and claims filed in its name.

High-Risk Obstetrical Practices . . . Know Enough to Stay Away

Doctor-shopping would be a whole lot easier if someone would profile the malpracticing obstetrician— that is, inventory the typical traits of obstetricians who incur high malpractice risk, either for what they do or for what they do not do. Well, someone has, and who better to have done so than a lawyer for the defense, who along with the doctor and the consumer is the other person most privy to the practices and actions that result in a charge of malpractice?

"Dunn's Rule." That's what Lee J. Dunn, Jr., J.D., a partner in the Boston firm of Dunn and Auton, calls this profile, based on his nearly twenty years of experience in medical malpractice suits, plus conversations with many other defense lawyers and plaintiffs' attorneys. "Hardly a scientific study," he freely admits, "but time after time experience has shown me and many others that the rule holds true." (Apparently consumers are not the only ones hungry for such an analysis: we caught up with Dunn not long after a presentation he made at an update on medicolegal issues in obstetrics and gynecology presented by the Harvard Medical School.)

According to Dunn, cases with significant verdicts or settlements tend to fall into at least one and usually two or more of the following categories:

1. "The physician is a graduate of a foreign medical school or, if trained in the U.S., is over 50 years of age and not board-certified." With foreign medical school graduates, Dunn says, the problem is not necessarily one of a poorer medical education, but more a matter of inability to communicate effectively in colloquial English. The issue of age and board-certification status, in his view, too often comes down to a lag in knowledge and skills—the newest practices and latest changes in obstetrics, "probably the fastest changing area of medicine."

2. "The cases occur in a community hospital," which does not have the advantages of a tertiary care hospital, with its medical residents ("one more guardian at the gate"), house officers, stringent peer review system, and other steps to help ensure quality, according to Dunn.

3. "Abuse of oxytocin [administered to induce or hasten labor]." When administered for other than sound clinical reasons, this practice, Dunn explains, can become more a matter of convenience for the physician than of medical necessity.

4. "Poor medical record-keeping," reflecting an overall sloppiness.

(continued)

5. "The physician delivers more than 300 babies a year." Two problems derive from this, the latest addition to Dunn's Rule: the practitioner is just "too busy" to give proper care and "too often delegates prenatal care to nurses or others who are not prepared for emergencies or complications that may arise."

Your Choices in Maternity Care Providers

While most pregnancies do not run a high risk of complications or carry a risk of negligent or improper care, your doctor's competence will have great impact on your *chances* of being malpracticed on. The fact is, most consumers spend more time selecting their roofer than they do choosing someone to provide their medical care. The earlier you start to shop for the right birth practitioner, the better. This way you have the time to approach the process from a consumerist perspective—ask the right questions, evaluate the answers, and choose among your various options. And an early start gives you enough leeway to change practitioners, if you desire, before the final stage of the journey: labor and delivery.

Choosing a birth practitioner isn't easy. It's a process filled with questions, both for the prospective provider and for yourself, but the right choice can save you heartbreak and money. After all, bad medical care costs much more than good medical care—it takes its toll on your health and your family, as well as on your pocketbook.

Obstetrician

The great majority of women choose an obstetrician-gynecologist for their birth practitioner; in fact, obstetricians deliver four out of every five babies born in this country. This doesn't necessarily mean that this is the choice for you. Most women do choose an ob-gyn because they want the "reassurance" that they believe only a medical specialist can give: that

45

any complication that arises can be "handled." But you should realize that the way many ob-gyns handle the vast majority of complications involves invasive, often risky procedures, not the least of which is surgery, such as cesarean sections. By the same token, if you would feel better knowing that you have access to the latest medical technology, then you will probably want an obstetrician for your primary maternity-care provider.

As in any medical specialty, the ob-gyn is a product of his medical education, which in this case entails a minimum of three years of specialty training (called a *residency*) in obstetrics and gynecology after medical school. At the heart of the ob-gyn residency is surgical training—somewhere around 75 percent of it, say Korte and Scaer in *A Good Birth, A Safe Birth.*

A particularly revealing account of one doctor's residency in obstetrics and gynecology at a major American hospital is *A Woman in Residence*, by Michelle Harrison, M.D. (New York: Random House, 1982). In her book Harrison describes the grueling hours of her residency: "I was in surgery seven hours from 7 a.m. until two in the afternoon. Usually there were a half dozen or more operations, and I'd make rounds in between or after." An indictment of medical education, as well as the maternity care system in this country, *A Woman in Residence* draws parallels between medical training and "brainwashing: Two major components are sleep deprivation and isolation from one's support system."

Obstetricians are the product of a system that, in the words of Korte and Scaer, "[believes] birth to be a time of highest risk to the baby." In such a view, the obstetrician's job is "to get the baby out as quickly as possible," and if this obligation opens the door to intervention in almost all births, so be it.

Many obstetricians are board-certified, meaning that they have completed postgraduate training in their field. In addition, they have passed an examination administered by the specialty board, a national board of professionals in that specialty field. A doctor who passes the board examination is given the status of *Diplomate*. Also, most board-certified doctors become members of their medical specialty societies, and any doctor who meets the full requirements for membership is called a *Fellow* of the society and may use the designation. In the case of an ob-gyn, the initials "FACOG" after a doctor's name denotes that she is a Fellow of the American College of Obstetricians and Gynecologists.

In its most basic sense, board certification indicates that a physician has completed a course of study in accordance with the established educational standards of one or more of the twenty-three member boards of the American Board of Medical Specialties, a Chicago-based independent regulatory body. Board certification has been called a minimum standard of excellence and nothing more. True, paper certification does not produce professional excellence. On the other hand, although there are some inferior doctors who somehow manage to become board-certified, and there are some excellent doctors without board certification, board certification is a good sign that the person is up to date on the procedures, theories, and success–failure rates in the specialty. Our earlier caveat regarding medical specialties is important to repeat here: *Be aware that a licensed physician may practice any specialty and call himself a specialist in a particular field, whether or not the physician is actually board-certified in that specialty.*

To verify the credentials of any obstetrician claiming board certification, contact the American Board of Obstetrics and Gynecology (see p. 22 for the address and telephone number).

If the obstetrician is a doctor of osteopathy (D.O.) rather than an M.D. (see p. 50), contact the American Osteopathic Board of Obstetrics and Gynecology, Osteopathic Medical Center, 5200 S. Ellis Street, Chicago, IL 60615; telephone 1- 312-947-3000.

──────── *Family Practitioner*

A relatively new specialty, family practice is concerned with the total health care of the individual and the family and not limited to any age, sex, organ system, or disease entity. The family practitioner (FP) has three years of training following medical school, including a minimum of three months of obstetrics and gynecology. Because the FP is what's called a primary care physician and can provide comprehensive care to the entire family, many pregnant women like the continuity of

Keeping Your Gynecologist on as Obstetrician

If you have already established a good rapport and trusting relationship with a gynecologist (if you have one) and you are satisfied with her competence and credentials, perhaps you would be content with the quick hat change that transforms her into your obstetrician—that is, if she continues to maintain an obstetric side to the business and hasn't joined the reputed legions of ob-gyns leaving the baby-delivering side.

But before you make your final decision, schedule a consultation to discuss some of the issues pertinent to obstetric care. Compare your gynecologist's viewpoints with your own on topics such as hospital versus birthing center, high-tech interventions in pregnancy—for example, routine ultrasound or amniocentesis, labor induction, anesthesia and drugs during delivery, and so on—and the other issues that will help you decide whether you can work together for the nine months it takes to have a baby. And consider your other options.

care this doctor offers. Korte and Scaer describe the philosophical orientation to birth and interventions: "Family practitioners view birth as a normal process. Because they take care of newborns just as pediatricians do, they often see the complications from interventions. They view intervention in labor and delivery as risky and see themselves as skillfully using interventions only when necessary."

Of course, not every FP has obstetrical experience. You will want to find out from the outset not only whether he has any experience at all, but what proportion of the doctor's practice is obstetrics, how many babies the doctor has delivered, whether there were complications, and if so, what, and whether he has handled high-risk pregnancies.

To verify the credentials of an M.D. purporting to be board-certified in family practice—although, remember, that doesn't mean that the doctor has done anything more than a brief stint in obstetrics training—contact the American Board of

Maternal and Fetal Medicine

Maternal and fetal medicine is a subspecialty of obstetrics. At last count, there were 560 board-certi-fied maternal and fetal medicine specialists (also called perinatolo-gists) nationwide. (Remember: to be board-certified the doctor must have completed postgraduate training and passed an oral and written exam.) Any obstetrician who hangs out this shingle may have received this additional training in high-risk pregnancies—but may not have, and instead is just enjoying the priv-ilege of self-proclaiming a specialty. Double-check those credentials!

A pregnancy is deemed high risk when you have a preexisting medical condition—such as cystic fi-brosis, diabetes, heart disease, or high blood pressure—before you be-come pregnant. In this case, your regular physician will probably rec-ommend that you receive your ma-ternity care from such a specialist. Or, even if you are healthy and have no preexisting serious medical prob-lems, you may develop complica-tions over the course of your preg-nancy and be referred to a maternal medicine specialist, if your doctor or midwife—whomever you've chosen for your maternity care—feels this is necessary.

Because specialty care is usually more expensive and certainly more high tech, you should ask your doc-tor a couple of key questions before you see a specialist:

Why do I have to see a specialist? Ask your doctor for a good explana-tion of what he thinks is wrong with you. Ask for—demand, if neces-sary—a complete and understand-able, point-by-point diagnostic por-trait. Going to a specialist should not be a casual next step routinely taken, whatever the medical situa-tion.

Why this particular specialist? Why Dr. A and not Dr. B or even Dr. C? Is A the best person for the job? Are you being sent because Dr. A is an excellent representative of her profession? Or is it because Dr. A and your doctor are old buddies who have an arrangement, each recom-mending the other?

You should come away from this dialogue *confident* that legitimate need and competence are the rea-sons for the referral.

M.D.'s and D.O.'s
What's the Difference?

Osteopathy, the often forgotten branch of mainstream medical care, is by no means insignificant in numbers of practitioners: twenty-eight thousand in the United States. Overshadowed by allopathic medicine and the one-half million M.D.'s who practice it, osteopathy is frequently ignored, partly as a result of the public perception that the M.D. is the sole torchbearer for traditional medicine. This simply is not true. Both osteopathy and allopathy claim scientifically accepted methods of diagnosis and treatment as their basis. D.O.'s and M.D.'s are essentially the same, except for a notable difference in philosophy and, to a lesser extent, practice habits. If traditional medicine can be neatly categorized into two basic approaches—focus on the patient versus focus on the patient's disease—osteopathy stresses the former.

In brief, D.O.'s, or doctors of osteopathy, are fully licensed physicians and surgeons who hold that the body is an interrelated system. The practitioners are called *osteopaths* because they emphasize the role of bones, muscles, and joints of the body—the musculoskeletal system—in a person's well-being.

Given this emphasis, manipulation and hands-on diagnosis and treatment are mainstays of osteopathic practice and are, in short, what distinguish D.O.'s from M.D.'s. Generally, compared to M.D.'s, D.O.'s *tend* to be more holistic in their approach to care, *tend*—at least at first—not to order a full battery of tests for diagnostic purposes but instead rely on a more selective range, and *tend* to utilize manipulation before drugs and surgery. However, while it is true that D.O.'s underscore the body's natural ability to heal itself, they also utilize the usual bag of medical tricks, all the recognized procedures and modern technologies, including drugs, radiation, and surgery.

Whether one becomes a D.O. or an M.D., the route of medical training is basically the same. In matters of licensing, D.O.'s hold the same unlimited practice rights as M.D.'s in all fifty states and the District of Columbia, and can admit and treat patients in both osteopathic and allopathic hospitals and clinics. There are nearly two hundred designated osteopathic hospitals in the United States, which provide special osteopathic care in addition to general medical-surgical services. But more likely than not, D.O.'s practice alongside M.D.'s in allopathic facilities.

Most D.O.'s are generalists, but some have additional training and qualifications and work in specialized fields, which, except insofar as the basic approach to care differs, resemble allopathic specialties. Ob-

(continued)

stetrics and gynecology is one of the seventeen areas of certification recognized by the American Osteopathic Association (AOA), a trade organization similar to the American Medical Association.

Bear in mind that, as with the M.D., the osteopathic practitioner can self-designate a specialty: without the benefit of additional training and without the benefit of certifying credentials from an AOA-sanctioned board. To check on the credentials of a D.O., you will want to contact the certifying board for her specialty (see below).

Family Practice, 2228 Young Drive, Lexington, Kentucky 40505; telephone 1-606-269-5626.

To verify the credentials of a D.O./family practitioner, contact the American Osteopathic Board of General Practice, 330 East Algonquin Road, #2, Arlington Heights, Illinois 60005; telephone 1-708-635-8477. Again, credentials in this specialty indicate only that the doctor has spent some time (but maybe not a lot, or enough for you) in obstetrics training.

Your choices in nonphysician providers include the following:

Certified Nurse-Midwife

Women having babies historically were attended by other women until the medicalization of childbirth succeeded in discrediting the practice of midwifery. Although the American College of Nurse-Midwives (ACNM) held its first general meeting in 1955 and was recognized by the international association of midwives the next year, it was not until the early 1970s that the American College of Obstetricians and Gynecologists officially endorsed the practice of nurse-midwifery. Today, approximately forty-two hundred certified nurse-midwives practice in all fifty states.

A certified nurse-midwife is a registered nurse who has completed at least one year of obstetric training in an approved graduate midwifery program, demonstrated clinical experi-

51

ence, and passed the national certification examination given by the American College of Nurse-Midwives. Then she must obtain a license or permit to practice in the state where she intends to work. Indeed, all but a few states require that a nurse applying to practice as a nurse-midwife hold current ACNM certification. The states that do not recognize or require certification by the ACNM for licensure are Maine, Minnesota, Missouri, Oregon, and Virginia.

Nurse-midwives limit their practice to managing the maternity care of women whose progress through pregnancy and labor and delivery is normal and uncomplicated, and also provide postpartum care to both the mother and the newborn baby. The certified nurse-midwife is trained to recognize the signs of an abnormal situation in either pregnancy or childbirth and to refer to a specialist, when necessary. For many pregnant women, the enormous appeal of nurse-midwifery lies in its noninterventional approach to childbirth; its emphasis on helping educate the woman to assume more control over the birth process by stressing childbirth education and prenatal care; and its affirmation of psychological as well as medical support of the woman. If you do not want or need a high-tech childbirth, nurse-midwifery is worth more than a second glance.

On the other hand, just a quick look at state laws nationwide governing the scope of practice of nurse-midwifery reveals disparity and diversity in what nurse-midwives can do. We can say with certainty, however, that the vast majority of states require practicing nurse-midwives to have written agreements, or contracts, with supervising physicians and/or health care facilities. This doesn't mean that in every state the physician must be in *direct* supervision—that is, right on the spot—during pregnancy and childbirth; it means only that a written protocol must be established regarding the extent of an obstetrician's supervision of the cases.

As to what nurse-midwives can and cannot do, it is up to you to find out the situation in your particular state. Alabama, for example, specifies that beech presentation, multiple pregnancies, and forceps delivery are outside the nurse-midwife's scope of practice. In similar wording, California's law prohibits her from engaging in "artificial, forcible, or mechanical means, specifically the use of forceps, vacuum extractors, and cesarean section." Also in California the ratio of nurse-midwife to supervising physician cannot exceed three to one. The Idaho law accentuates the positive in its wording and allows the nurse-midwife to "utilize standing orders to start [intravenous] infusions, administer analgesics, and administer oxytocin [to induce or hasten labor] in the third stage of labor, . . . give local, paracervical, or pudendal anesthesia, . . . perform episiotomies and repairs" and so on. In some states, nurse-midwives even have authority to write prescriptions. Call your state nurse licensing board (see Appendix D) for more information on your state's laws.

Nurse-midwives practice in a variety of settings—county hospitals, private hospitals, neighborhood health centers, private physicians' offices, and birthing centers—but the majority of births (85 percent, according to the ACNM) attended by nurse-midwives occur in hospitals, 11 percent in birthing centers, and 4 percent in homes.

To find a certified nurse-midwife in your area, contact the American College of Nurse-Midwives, 1522 K Street, N.W., Suite 1000, Washington, D.C. 20005; telephone 1-202-289-4379.

You can also call a university near you to see whether it has a nurse-midwifery program (some do) or you can contact certified childbirth education programs (see p. 136).

Lay Midwife

Unlike the nurse-midwife, the lay midwife practices in a home setting; she is not a licensed nurse and does not have formal training in obstetrics. Instead, in most cases she has learned by doing; she has attended births, usually first as an apprentice to more experienced midwives, then as the primary birth attendant. Because lay midwives acquire their skills through observation and experience, they often call themselves "empirical" midwives. Traditionally, they assisted in areas where medical care was unavailable, and until recently their numbers were dwindling. Fortunately for women desiring this option, however, there has been a general reemergence of the practice of lay midwifery. According to a September 1988 *American Journal of Public Health* article, which talks about an "extensive grassroots movement of lay midwives committed to quality of care," a number of factors are responsible for the comeback:

> questioning of medical domination of childbirth, demanding the right by childbearing women to choose place of birth and birth practitioner, searching for safe alternatives to hospital births, worrying over escalating childbirth costs, the general shifting of specific services away from hospitals, [and] desiring of more natural and woman-centered childbirth experiences.

State laws concerning the legal status and practice of lay midwifery are considerably diverse. A national survey by the article's authors netted these findings. As of July 1987:

- Ten states prohibit the practice of lay midwifery: Alabama, California, Colorado, Connecticut, Hawaii, Maryland, North Carolina, Pennsylvania, West Virginia, and Wisconsin.
- Five states have "grandmother clauses," which allow lay midwifery under repealed statutes only: Delaware, Illinois, Kentucky, Rhode Island, and Virginia.
- Four states and the District of Columbia have laws that allow lay midwifery practice, but no licenses have been issued in recent years: Georgia, Minnesota, Mississippi, and New Jersey.
- Ten states explicitly permit or regulate the practice: Alaska, Arizona, Arkansas, Florida, Louisiana, New Hampshire, New Mexico, South Carolina, Texas, and Washington.
- The remaining twenty-one states—Idaho, Indiana, Iowa, Kansas, Maine, Massachusetts, Michigan, Missouri, Montana, Nebraska, Nevada, New York, North Dakota, Ohio, Oklahoma, Oregon, South Dakota, Tennessee, Utah, Vermont, and Wyoming—have no laws pertaining to lay midwifery, and in some cases the legal status is unclear. This is not to say, of course, that lay midwives are not practicing in these states, just that if they are, they are practicing "outside the regulatory auspices of state government."

In those states that explicitly allow lay midwifery, the minimum requirements for licensing and the scope of practice (any prohibitions and restrictions) vary. New Mexico, for example, issues three types of registration permits to lay midwives and requires four recommendations and certification in both adult and newborn cardiopulmonary resuscitation (CPR). In Texas, every lay midwife must register with the county where she resides or practices and must perform certain duties, including screening pregnant women for syphilis and their newborns for various diseases. Lay midwives in Louisiana are required to renew their licenses annually and at that time demonstrate current CPR certification and show evidence of ten hours of continuing education. All states specify that all midwives confine their practice to low-risk, or "normal and uncomplicated," pregnancies, and some require at least one prenatal examination by a physician even though the woman is working with a lay midwife.

From just this small sampling, you can see that state laws range all over the place, and, frankly, legislation is in such a state of flux that it is hard to make any certain pronouncements. Where can you find out the *current* legal status of the practice of lay midwifery in your state? Contact your state health department (see Appendix E). If you do not get the information you need there, you can try your state nurse licensing board (Appendix D) or medical licensing board (see Appendix B), although remember that in a number of states lay midwifery is frowned on if not outright outlawed.

Pennsylvania is an interesting case in point. So determined are the lay midwives there to gain legal recognition that in a 1990 rally at the state capitol hundreds of Amish and Mennonites broke from their tradition of shunning political activity and showed up in support of proposals to permit midwives who are not registered nurses. The issue has struck a nerve with these religious communities, which describe the practice of midwifery as an integral part of their life-style and heritage.

We have stressed the importance of checking the training and credentials of any birth practitioner you are considering, and the same holds true for lay midwives—especially since their training and experience vary. If you choose a lay midwife because you both agree that your pregnancy seems "normal and uncomplicated," be sure to have a medical backup for any problems that may arise.

Infant and Maternal Mortality Rates (1985)

Infant Mortality[1]

Hospital	Nonhospital	
10.5/1,000	21/1,000	*Physician*
5.2/1,000	4.7/1,000	*Midwife*
22.1/1,000	18.1/1,000	*Other*[3]

Maternal Mortality[2]

7.8/100,000

1. *Source:* National Center for Health Statistics, National Linked Birth and Infant Death File, 1985.
2. Unspecified as to particular setting or practitioner. *Source:* National Center for Health Statistics, National Linked Birth and Infant Death File, 1985.
3. Attendant not specified on birth certificate. Could be nurse, family member, EMT, police officer, cab driver, friend, clergy, or the like.

Again, certified childbirth education programs may be able to refer you to midwives in your community. Of course, don't forget the recommendations of friends or others, but be sure to follow up with a lot of questions.

Before we go on to the face-to-face interview and agenda of questions, a few more thoughts are appropriate here concerning the medical management of a pregnancy. Whichever kind of practitioner you choose, bear in mind that in dealing with the system you are swimming against a current of dogma that Ann Oakley in *Women Confined: Towards a Sociology of Childbirth* (New York: Schocken Books, 1980) calls the "medical frame of reference." Two particular features of this are the idea that "doctor knows best" (that is, doctors know more about having babies than women do) and the fact that pregnant women have had limited status in the overall medical management of their pregnancies. Both aspects are a part of the whole picture Oakley calls "medical control of reproduction," and too often "conflict between reproducer as expert and doctor as expert" results.

Should you choose a physician, any conflict *can* have a favorable outcome or even be prevented if you have information and conviction. You can further strengthen your position by finding a supportive doctor who will recognize that you are an equal partner in any and all medical decisions regarding your pregnancy and your baby. Yes, there are doctors out there who will work with you on an equal partnership basis. You just need to know what to ask.

In 1983, the People's Medical Society produced a statement, a Code of Practice, that we believe each doctor should subscribe to. Ask the doctors you're considering for your birth practitioner to review the Code of Practice and tell you whether they will apply it to your care. Although an affirmative answer won't tell you whether the doctor embraces the premise that pregnancy is a healthy, normal condition, the Code of Practice will help you find a doctor with whom you can enjoy active participation and decision-making power in your own health care.

The People's Medical Society Code of Practice

I will assist you in finding information resources, support groups, and health care providers to help you maintain and improve your health. When you seek my care for specific problems, I will abide by the following Code of Practice:

Office Procedures

1. I will post or provide a printed schedule of my fees for office visits, procedures, tests, and surgery, and provide itemized bills.

2. I will provide certain hours each week when I will be available for nonemergency telephone consultation.

3. I will schedule appointments to allow the necessary time to see you with minimal waiting. I will promptly report test results to you and return phone calls.

57

4. I will allow and encourage you to bring a friend or relative into the examining room with you.

5. I will facilitate your getting your medical and hospital records, and will provide you with copies of your test results.

———— *Choice in Diagnosis and Treatment*

6. I will let you know your prognosis, including whether your condition is terminal or will cause disability or pain, and will explain why I believe further diagnostic activity or treatment is necessary.

7. I will discuss with you diagnostic, treatment, and medication options for your particular problem (including the option of no treatment), and describe in understandable terms the risk of each alternative, the chances of success, the possibility of pain, the effect on your functioning, the number of visits each would entail, and the cost of each alternative.

8. I will describe my qualifications to perform the proposed diagnostic measures or treatments.

9. I will let you know of organizations, support groups, and medical and lay publications that can assist you in understanding, monitoring, and treating your problem.

10. I will not proceed until you are satisfied that you understand the benefits and risks of each alternative and I have your agreement on a particular course of action.

———— *Evaluating Your Practitioner: Question, Question, Question*

If you are like most women, you will choose a physician as your birth practitioner. (Physicians were present at 97 percent of all deliveries in 1989, according to a Health Insurance Association of America survey—midwives, at merely 3 percent.) So we will call your birth attendant a doctor.

Word-of-mouth—getting a few good recommendations from family members, friends, and neighbors—is a good way to begin your search. You will want to follow up these recommendations with some sleuthing of your own.

A doctor referral service, usually operated by the local medical society or a local hospital, can be another source of names of health care providers. Not necessarily our first choice, such services give out only the names of doctors who are members of the society or are on the hospital staff. Lest you attach altruistic motives to the physician referral services, which approximately two-thirds of all community hospitals run, bear in mind that the economic incentive is to fill empty hospital beds—precisely what doctors do for hospitals. In such a setup, clearly the doctors most popular with the hospital *and* its referral service are the ones who maintain a brisk admission tempo. Another major drawback to either medical-society- or hospital-sponsored services is that neither will comment on the ability and competence of physicians other than perhaps to mention their board certifications.

Newspaper advertisements, even the seemingly innocuous announcement of the opening of a new practice, may either be useful or have dubious value, too. Ask yourself why the doctor is advertising: To attract patients because he is just out of medical school? Or is in a highly competitive and glutted market? Or has he just moved in from a state where his license was revoked, and he needs new victims? Furthermore, just because a doctor says he specializes in a certain area of medicine does not mean the doctor actually took any advanced training in it; a doctor can practice in any specialty area he chooses.

We have already discussed how a doctor's credentials—where educated, what specialty training and certification—and competence can be checked by preliminary research, and certainly you *should* feel confident in your birth practitioner's expertise and technical skills. But you must also trust that person, feel comfortable bringing up questions and concerns, and assure yourself that he will work with you and your partner to help you have the pregnancy and childbirth experiences you desire. All the best credentials and board certifications do not guarantee that the doctor will be communicative or that he will be interested in your preferences. That's why we suggest a get-acquainted visit.

The Get-Acquainted Visit

The object is to determine if you and the doctor are right for each other. When you telephone for an appointment, be sure to tell the receptionist that you want to arrange a get-acquainted visit. If the doctor refuses, go on to the next doctor on your list. Be aware that some doctors charge for a get-acquainted visit and some do not. Some busy doctors with established practices may not want to give their time away, while other doctors are eager for new business and willing to waive even a nominal charge for a get-acquainted visit. If the environment in your community is competitive and doctors are clamoring for business, the get-acquainted visit becomes even more of a selling point. As one practice management consultant tells doctors wondering whether or not to charge, "Count the holes in your appointment calendar." The doctor who agrees to a get-acquainted visit may be more consumer-oriented than other doctors, but she may also be motivated solely by economic considerations.

The first thing you want to observe is the doctor's office setup and staff. Most offices have a receptionist who will greet you and ask you to complete a few forms for their records. Ask the receptionist to brief you on the particulars regarding making appointments, telephoning the doctor, getting prescription refills, and obtaining copies of your medical records.

A first-time visit will probably run ten to fifteen minutes, so you need to have your questions ready and make the minutes count. Some of the initial questions you should raise can be answered by the receptionist (maybe even over the telephone); others the doctor must answer. Pay particular attention to the doctor's manner and attitude as she answers your questions. Is the doctor addressing the heart of your questions and answering in a forthright manner? Or is there an impatience or hesitation?

■ *How long has the doctor been in practice? What are the doctor's credentials—medical degree, board certification, and other specialized and/or postgraduate education—and hospital affiliations? What is the doctor's record of continuing education?*

If the doctor is not on staff at the hopsital of your choosing, or if she (as is often the case in larger cities) delivers babies at more than one hospital, each with a routine and protocol all its own, then perhaps a better course of action for you is first to choose the hospital (see p. 67), and then shop around for a doctor who admits there.

■ *Will the doctor deliver your baby at home?*

If you are interested in this option (see p. 78), ask this question right away, but realize that few doctors, especially obstetricians, will stray far from the hospital's high-tech medical equipment.

■ *How much does maternity care (normal prenatal care and delivery) cost? What does the fee cover? Does the doctor have a fee schedule or payment plan? Is your insurance coverage accepted?*

A doctor who will openly discuss her fees may be more willing to discuss other aspects of your medical care. A Health Insurance Association of America survey found that a normal pregnancy and delivery cost $4,334 in 1989, although that figure varied regionally across the United States: the highest costs in the Northeast ($4,456) and the lowest ($4,149) in the Midwest. Each delivery rang up an average of $1,492 on the delivering physician's cash register (tote up an average of $994 for a midwife). Make sure any fee includes office visits and routine lab work (urinalysis, blood tests for protein and sugar levels, and antibody serum for the Rh factor), and perhaps even the follow-up visit six weeks after delivery. Doctors often require full payment by the seventh month; meanwhile, you must wait until after the baby is born for insurance reimbursement. As to insurance coverage, the Health Insurance Association of

61

America survey found that in 1989 private insurers covered maternity costs, at least in part, for 64 percent of women.

■■■ *What is the scheduled length of appointments? How often must you schedule visits? How long is the typical wait?*

A quick glance around the waiting room should give you a good idea of whether the doctor overbooks—that is, crowds too many appointments into too short a time frame, the inevitable outcome being rushed and hurried consultations and/or long waits. Except for emergencies that interrupt even the best-organized office routines and most caring practices, there's no excuse for this, least of all greed.

■■■ *Is the practice solo or group? If group, do all the doctors share the same obstetrical philosophy and practices? Can prenatal visits be arranged on a rotation basis with each doctor in the group?*

The solo practice is almost a vanishing breed, especially in obstetrics. While a group practice takes the pressure off the individual doctor's practice and reduces the work load on each doctor so that, hypothetically at least, your doctor can spend more time with you, the potential downside is an overcrowded waiting room due to overbooking, and the feeling that you are receiving assembly-line, fragmented medical care. You also run the risk of establishing a good rapport with one doctor, only to have a member of the group you have never met or with whom you are uncomfortable attend you on delivery day. So not only is it important for you to meet every doctor in the practice, but you should be able to request—and have your own doctor agree—that a particular doctor in the group *not* attend your labor and delivery.

■■■ *Does the doctor have a midwife on her staff?*

Recognizing the knowledge, expertise, and understanding that a midwife can bring to pregnancy and childbirth, increasing numbers of physicians—although still a minority of practices—are adding midwives to their staffs.

■ *Do medical residents or interns assist in the doctor's practice?*

The supervision of doctors-in-training is not uncommon, but again the problem is that you may find yourself being treated by someone you don't know, someone who is in essence an apprentice and, therefore, lacks the experience of the doctor you *chose.*

■ *Does the doctor endorse "prepared childbirth"?*

While you don't necessarily have to discuss at this time all the various prenatal education programs designed to teach expectant parents about pregnancy, the stages of normal labor, and pain management during birth, you can at least get a sense of whether the doctor supports even the notion of courses in childbirth. Not all do.

■ *Will the doctor endorse the People's Medical Society Code of Practice?*

The Code of Practice is a useful gauge of the doctor's willingness to accept you as a health care consumer rather than a patient, as a person who requires information and choices to make decisions rather than a person who accepts what's given to her.

Know the Pregnancy and Birth You Want

Not every one of the following considerations may be important to you, but it is important to know what you want, then find out whether the doctor's philosophy or method of practice is compatible with your desires. Ask the doctor:

● *What method of childbirth preparation do you prefer?*

● *What prenatal tests/procedures do you recommend?*

● *Do you encourage or allow the father's presence, both in prenatal visits and during labor and birth? What about during a cesarean section? A major victory this one, the presence of the father in the delivery room, but some doctors and hos-*

pitals still refuse. The father as coach, supporter, and reporter is a viable member of the obstetrical *team* and integral to family-centered birth.

- *Do you encourage or allow siblings to visit the baby in the hospital where you practice?*

- *Do you encourage breast-feeding? Do you allow the woman to breast-feed immediately following birth, while she's still in the delivery room (assuming both mother and baby are healthy)?* Doctors usually are not experts in breast-feeding, especially not in the area of "how to" advice, but should you choose this feeding method, you want to know that the doctor will be supportive.

- *What is your cesarean-section rate?* (Although the nation's rate is around 25 percent, suggested figures range from 7.6 to 12 percent.) *What indications or criteria do you follow? What is your position on the "once a cesarean, always a cesarean" maxim?*

- *In what percentage of your patients do you induce labor? Are episiotomies routine in your obstetrical practice? What about forceps delivery or vacuum extraction—in what percentage of the births in your practice are these methods used?* Numbers here are hard to come by. However, according to guidelines issued by the American College of Obstetricians and Gynecologists, 1 to 4 percent of births may result in the use of forceps, an acceptable percentage in the college's opinion.

- *Do you routinely use drugs—analgesic or anesthetic—in the management of pain during labor? If so, what are the most common ones?*

- *Do you routinely require restraints and/or straps during delivery? Stirrups?*

- *Do you encourage women to try different birthing positions?*

- *Is continuous fetal heart-rate monitoring a routine procedure in childbirths you attend?*

The Birth Plan

If you can find a doctor willing to go along with the majority of your concerns and choices, then you're doing well. And you're doing even better if you can draw up a written agreement, often called a birth plan, and convince the doctor to sign it and abide by it. A device advocated by many childbirth educators and consumer advocates, this checklist of preferences and instructions works best as a reminder to the doctor of the important care issues discussed and treatment options agreed on *long before* the labor and delivery, that time when even the best-laid plans can fall victim to an oblivious doctor and unyielding hospital employees. Labor and delivery is not the optimum time to be dickering over details!

In *Birthrights* (New York: Pantheon, 1984), Sally Inch cautions against viewing the birth plan as "a way of assuming some sort of control over events once the mother is in the hospital." Only a convenient reminder and not a contract, a birth plan is most valuable prenatally when, she says, it "serves to identify the basic philosophies and flexibility of the care givers and to reveal any important areas of disagreement at a time when it is still possible for the mother to change her birth attendants."

You will find a sample birth plan in Appendix F. Review it with your partner and your doctor, and modify it where necessary to reflect your preferences and any negotiated points on which you and your doctor agree.

Ask the doctor to keep a copy of the birth plan in your medical record at his office *and* send a copy to the hospital or birthing center where you expect to deliver. Of course, your copy will be with you when you go to the hospital. Refer to it, wave it around if necessary—especially after changes in staff during your labor—but don't let it replace cooperative, effective dialogue with your doctor.

Know Your Rights

You do have certain rights as a consumer of any kind of medical care. Knowing what these rights are and finding a

65

practitioner who views you as a partner and acknowledges these rights undoubtedly will help you have the kind of pregnancy and childbirth you want. Childbirth educator Valmai Howe Elkins, in her book *The Rights of the Pregnant Parent* (New York: Schocken Books, 1980), lists six "basic human rights" that have not been legally recognized, but that nonetheless she considers the rights of every pregnant woman and her partner. They are

1. the right to a supportive doctor;
2. the right to a healthy baby;
3. the right to childbirth education;
4. the right to a shared birth experience;
5. the right to childbirth with dignity; and
6. the right to family-centered maternity care.

For more information on your rights, we have included in Appendixes G and H documents addressing the rights and the responsibilities of the patient and the pregnant patient.

Always remember: You have the right to participate in any and all decisions involving your well-being and the health of your unborn child. Unmistakable medical emergencies are the only exceptions, and even then it's possible for you and your doctor to have come to a prior agreement about the "what if" and "then this."

CHAPTER FOUR

Choosing a Birth Setting

The type of childbirth experience you have depends very much on where you decide to have your baby. Some women desire a setting as similar to home as possible, where the sights are familiar and the routine flexible and undemanding. For others, only the traditional medical environment will do, complete with clinical specialists and the latest medical and obstetrical equipment—a setting where personal touches and first-name camaraderie often take a backseat to hospital protocol and clinical precision.

Clearly, where birth settings are concerned, different strokes for different folks.

The Hospital

Actually, depending on the hospital, you may have a choice of two sites: a standard delivery room (really a suite because labor, delivery, and recovery are in separate rooms) and a birthing room. If the mention of the former conjures up a roomful of mysterious machinery, cold-metal furnishings, blindingly bright lights, and white-garbed and masked people, you're right. Welcome to the conventional delivery room, home of all the high-tech equipment and interventionist procedures that have given modern obstetrics the reputation it has. And certainly they are a blessing if a problem occurs.

67

A delivery there is often a surgical procedure—a vaginal delivery with episiotomy and perhaps forceps or a cesarean section—or a "technological event," as Harrison describes it in *A Woman in Residence*. Women deliver in such a setting out of necessity as well as choice. For some women with problems—chronic illness, serious prenatal complications, and the like—the delivery room is the safest option; other women, with no problems at all, desire the reassurance that they believe only high-tech surroundings can give and so they choose the traditional setting. Or perhaps they want a hospital with a reputation in, say, neonatal (newborn) intensive care, so they are compelled to choose a large hospital, maybe even a university medical center, that offers such specialized care.

Whatever your own personal motivation, similar to shopping for the right birth practitioner, the key here is to choose a hospital that will help you assume an active role in your labor and delivery, and, of course, to continue to negotiate with your doctor for agreement on those options that are important to you. Just realize that you are likely to be more restricted in your choices in the conventional delivery room than anywhere else, and don't kid yourself—the rate of interventions and invasive procedures is usually quite high at most traditional hospitals. In choosing a hospital, especially the traditional route within this setting, the question to ask yourself is: Does your condition warrant high-tech medical intervention? Remember, such medical technology is best used only when appropriate to you. It should *not* be employed because the doctor's attitude is that all technology is good, or because the hospital routine demands it, or just because such technology exists. Every intervention carries some element of risk. It's up to you ultimately to weigh the risks to yourself and your baby. The longer you stay in a hospital and the more interventions proffered are factors that raise your risk of acquiring iatrogenic (doctor-produced) illness. For example, a surgical-site infection following a cesarean section or an adverse reaction to an anesthetic drug is not an uncommon iatrogenic outcome.

A birthing room, as mentioned above, is the other option within the hospital setting. Because a number of hospitals allow single-room maternity care—that is, the woman and her partner remain in place for labor, delivery, *and* recovery—the birthing room is usually a private room decorated to look as home*like* as possible: a "regular" bed (although in most cases the bed converts to allow other birthing positions) and perhaps a rocking chair or an easy chair for the woman's partner. Some hospitals, in order to attract obstetric customers, have employed interior designers to choose the fabrics, carpeting, and wall hangings. The homey atmosphere is an illusion, however, in the sense that the room is equipped with emergency resuscitative and obstetric equipment and down the hall is the delivery suite—in short, mere footsteps away is access to the standard interventions: IV hookups, electronic fetal monitors, delivery table with stirrups, and the like. There is little hard evidence to confirm that using a birthing room results in fewer interventions, only the suggestion or perhaps the illusion that it may, but clearly such settings have proven to be satisfying alternatives for women seeking more personal childbirth experiences in a less formal and intimidating atmosphere. Not only do most hospitals have strict protocols for screening who uses their birthing rooms, but many hospitals have only a few birthing rooms (and maybe only one). All this means that not every woman who wants to deliver in a birthing room gets her wish.

Beyond the Fluff of Hospital Marketing Tactics: Is It Really Family-Centered?

Birth choices in labor and delivery do vary from hospital to hospital, with some offering a great deal of flexibility and a staff committed to a family-centered birth, and others merely adding the floral bedspread or using a particular shade of mauve throughout the maternity wing. Hospitals, it is true, have been quick to see where new profit and public relations opportunities lie. And if that means catering to women and treating them better, then so be it. Hospitals have co-opted these concepts and created versions and interpretations of their own. In fact, however, truly family-centered care takes into account and involves the social and psychological aspects of birth, not only the physical ones. It takes into account the woman's wishes concerning such diverse matters as her partner's presence in the delivery room, her preference for her own nightgown rather than the hospital-issued gown, her desire to breast-feed immediately following delivery, or her wish to have her other children visit her and the newborn.

So go beyond the advertisements and public relations hucksterism to find the hospital that truly offers the approach you're seeking. Policies and protocols, all marketed under the umbrella term *family-centered*, are different from one hospital to another, and not every claim is legitimate. The concept of "rooming-in" is a good example. In some hospitals, this means you have your baby with you twenty-four hours a day, and you may choose to use the nursery for short intervals—that's the standard definition, and that's what many women want. But there are plenty of hospitals that restrict the hours to the convenience of the hospital routine; they limit "rooming-in" to only the day or sometimes at night. What about the hospital that crows about its new birthing room when it merely has moved labor and delivery into one room but retained all the standard interventions? Or the hospital that simply permits fathers to be present during labor and delivery, but changes no other obstetric protocol or routine? Is this legitimately family-centered care or merely superficialities intended to lure unwary customers? Is this what you're looking for?

Probably not. So what are you going to do? You probably *can* find the childbirth experience you want in a hospital—you just may have to hunt around for the right one. And there is no way to know what a hospital is really like except by giving it a good once-over in person. Seeing is believing, and asking is even better. Find out in which hospitals your doctor has privileges. Check those out first, then look into others that interest you. Call and set up an appointment for a walk-through tour of the hospital's maternity unit—as big a marketing tool as obstetrics is, you should have no problem, but if you do, don't hesitate to call the hospital administrator.

Again, question, question, question:

■ *What is the cesarean-section rate for the hospital?*

The word is out: most medical experts note that the United States is in the midst of a cesarean-section crisis. The national average is approximately 25 percent, but that varies regionally—with highest rates in the Northeast and South, and lowest in the Midwest and West. By comparison, England has recently reached an 11 percent cesarean section rate, which British experts consider too high.

■ *What is the hospital's nosocomial infection rate? The maternity unit's nosocomial rate? The newborn nursery's infection rate?*

Nosocomial infections, a form of iatrogenic illness, are those infections acquired during hospitalization and produced by microorganisms that dwell with relative impunity in hospitals. In other words, you didn't have it when you came in, but you got it while you were there.

■ *What childbirth preparation methods (Lamaze, for example) are the staff familiar with?*

Even a signed, sealed, and delivered understanding hammered out through discussions and negotiations with your doctor can be rendered useless by unsympathetic nurses and other attendants. At the very least, look for familiarity with various childbirth methods, and at best, support and encouragement.

■ *What childbirth preparation classes does the hospital offer? When are they provided—any evening classes so that working couples can attend? Is the father included?*

■ *Can the father attend the birth? What about another coach such as a lay midwife, or another supportive person such as a doula?*

A doula is a lay woman, usually a mother herself, who stays close to the woman through childbirth and primarily soothes and touches but does not coach or provide medical assessments or care; instead, she talks to the woman about what is happening. An article in the *Ob. Gyn. News* (June 15–30, 1989) reported the findings of a small study on the impact of this old practice. According to one of the study investigators,

71

the presence of a lay woman providing continuous social support "can significantly lower the incidence of medical interventions, shorten labor, and reduce the chance of a prolonged hospital stay for the neonate."

■ *What percentage of women have routine obstetric interventions—IVs, enemas, preps, and episiotomies?*

Unlike cesarean rates, no good figures are available here for you to compare, but again—you're trying to determine how far hospital protocol leans toward such interventions. Are they "givens"?

■ *Does the hospital encourage varied and alternative birth positions? If so, what?*

■ *Are there any guarantees that the birthing room(s) won't be in use when you need one?*

■ *Can the father remain in the operating room should a cesarean section be necessary?*

■ *Are there "rooming-in" provisions? Can the baby remain with the mother at all times, if the mother wishes? How soon after birth can "rooming-in" start?*

Elkins's rule here, from *The Rights of the Pregnant Parent*, is that the typical family-centered hospital will return the baby to the mother four to eight hours following birth. If longer than twelve hours is the norm, you may find yourself dealing with inflexibility in other policies as well.

■ *Is breast-feeding immediately after birth (assuming both the mother and the baby are healthy) encouraged?*

Again, you can generally assume that an answer of "It's not allowed" or "Our schedule doesn't permit it" means there are other rigid policies.

72

■ *Is there open visiting for fathers? Can siblings under the age of twelve visit the mother in the hospital?*

The truly family-centered hospital will recognize that the earlier that sibling attachment starts, the stronger the bond.

■ *Is length of stay flexible? If the mother and baby are healthy, is an early leave permissible?*

And what if you want to stay longer—for instance, you have a young child at home and need the extra time in the hospital—will the hospital be able to accommodate your wishes? Because the hospital is a place for sick people and indeed is full of sick people, we hardly recommend that you and your baby stay any longer than absolutely necessary. Plus, you may find yourself footing the bill when your insurance company denies coverage for the extra day(s). Nevertheless, ask the question if that's your wish.

Don't forget to find out whether the hospital is in good standing with the Joint Commission on Accreditation of Healthcare Organizations (JCAHO), a voluntary organization that sets standards for hospitals and other health care facilities, conducts periodic on-site inspections, and accredits facilities in compliance. You can ask the hospital administrator, but you may not trust a hospital with quality problems and operating under a conditional accreditation status (that is, given a limited time frame to clean up its act) to tell you the truth. Our advice is to go straight to JCAHO, which pledged a few years back to be more forthcoming about disclosing the names of hospitals with such problems ("deficiencies," in JCAHO jargon): Joint Commission on Accreditation of Healthcare Organizations, 1 Renaissance Boulevard, Oakbrook Terrace, Illinois 60187; telephone 1-708-916-5600.

Alternative Settings

Family-centered care *within* the hospital setting is only one alternative to routine hospital birth practices. Another alternative, the product of nearly two decades of intense consumer pressure and competition among practitioners and hospitals for business, is the birth center, sometimes called a childbearing center. And, of course, there also is the option of home birth.

────── **The Birth Center**

According to a Health Insurance Association of America survey, less than 0.5 percent of births took place in birth centers in 1989, but exact figures are hard to come by. Although the numbers of births are relatively small there, it is accurate to say that the idea of delivery in a birth center enjoys a loyal following: obstetricians (although certainly a minority of them), nurse- and lay midwives, childbirth educators, and consumers alike championing the low complication and cesarean-section rates, safety, cost savings, and consumer satisfaction that many birth centers offer. True, the statistics tell the real story: the overwhelming majority of doctors still prefer the hospital, and indeed, physician resistance to birth centers has been substantial. Organized medicine and medical traditionalists—groups such as the American Academy of Pediatrics and the American College of Obstetricians and Gynecologists—discourage the use of birth centers, but with 132 freestanding (meaning nonhospital-based) birth centers operating in the United States as of 1990, they are a viable choice for the woman looking to take more responsibility for her health care during pregnancy and delivery and to have an unmedicated childbirth, free of high-tech interventions.

Developed by midwives believing it to be the best alternative to both hospital and home deliveries, the birth center ideally offers a home*like* environment, a relaxed, flexible atmosphere, and very little intervention in the birth process—a process viewed as family-centered and "normal," not usually high-risk and dangerous. Most freestanding birth centers are owned by physicians or certified nurse-midwives, with most of the care provided by certified nurse-midwives working in consultation with obstetric and pediatric specialists on twenty-four-hour call. Some centers operate under the aegis of hospitals, and others are operated by community health centers or nonprofit groups (but the latter are relatively few in number).

Birth centers are designed to provide maternity care to women judged to be at low risk of obstetric complications; therefore, you should expect a strict screening process at any birth center you choose. Even if you are accepted after an initial prenatal visit, the center may decide further along in your pregnancy, or even during labor if an emergency or serious complications arise, to refer you to a hospital for your delivery. Most birth center programs incorporate childbirth education classes, classes for siblings who want to attend the birth, and postpartum support groups. The father (or other support person) is expected to attend the birth and, therefore, should prepare at classes. The protocol at most centers is relaxed, with no routine IVs, enemas, or preps (shave), and the woman is free to eat and do just about anything she wants during the childbirth experience: stay at home as long as possible, walk around during labor, and try a number of different labor and delivery positions to find the best, most comfortable one. Stays are short, and although early pediatric care is given at the center, women are expected to arrange for more extensive pediatric care within the first few days after returning home.

A 1989 survey conducted by the National Association of Childbearing Centers showed that, for normal birth, birth centers offer a 35 to 47 percent savings over hospitals, depending on the length of stay. A similar analysis that same year, this one by the Health Insurance Association of America, found that birth centers charge $1,000 less per day than hospitals do. And most health insurance plans cover birth at birth centers (but be sure to check the specific coverage under your policy). The picture of birth centers, where costs are concerned, is rosy.

"But How Safe Are They?" Since the early 1970s, when birth centers first arrived on the scene, medical establishment types and others have expressed concern about the potential medical risks of childbirth outside the hospital. Even when the transfer time between birth center and nearby hospital involves mere minutes, an interval that birth center proponents say mirrors

the time it takes a hospital to prepare for an emergency pro-cedure anyway, questions of safety remained, primarily be-cause of a lack of adequate research into outcomes. Although favorable, early studies of birth centers have been small.

However, a large-scale national study—the first of its kind—called the National Birth Center Study and published in the *New England Journal of Medicine* (December 28, 1989) has gone far in quelling much of the doubt about birth centers as safe alternatives to hospital childbirth for women judged to be at low risk of obstetric complications. After analyzing the ex-perience of 11,814 women admitted for labor and delivery at eighty-four freestanding birth centers from mid-1985 through 1987, the study concludes:

> [Birth] centers offer a safe and acceptable alternative to hospital confinement for selected pregnant women, partic-ularly those who have previously had children. . . . Few innovations in health service promise lower cost, greater availability, and a high degree of satisfaction with a com-parable degree of safety. The results of this study suggest that modern birth centers can identify women who are at low risk for obstetric complications and can care for them in a way that provides these benefits.

Specifically, the study found the following:

- About one in every six women admitted to participating birth centers was transferred to a hospital—more than half of the transfers for slow or stalled labor—with first-time mothers four times more likely to be transferred than women with children.

- The overall cesarean-section rate in the study population was a low 4.4 percent. (Although the study did not make direct comparisons, this rate is approximately half that reported in two published studies of hospital births in comparable low-risk populations.)

- Safety, as measured by maternal and infant mortality, was similar to that of university and community hospitals mea-sured in other studies. There were no maternal deaths, and the total infant mortality rate was 1.3 per 1,000 births (a rate similar to that reported in large studies of low-risk hospital births).

- The vast majority of women in the study reported that they would recommend the center to their friends and would return to the birth center for subsequent births.

Shopping for a Birth Center: Is It Licensed? Is It Accredited?

A majority, but not all, of the birth centers in the United States participated in the National Birth Center Study. Consequently, the researchers warn there is a chance that "the birth centers included . . . may be safer than those not included [in the study]," especially because fewer of the nonparticipating centers are licensed or accredited. Clearly this means that the wise consumer will rigorously examine the birth center before deciding to deliver there—including a walk-through tour such as we suggested you do with the hospital, and extensive questioning. To find a reputable birth center, you'll want to know:

▬ *Is the birth center freestanding—that is, nonhospital-based—and nonprofit? If not, under what arrangement with what hospital or other group does the center operate?*

These questions have to do with the issue of potential conflict of interest, the sort of you-scratch-my-back approach that more and more medical professionals are getting into *and* that more and more critics (even within the field) are decrying.

▬ *Does the center provide prenatal, childbirth, and postpartum care and education?*

▬ *Is there a community-based board of advisers? Who and what (consumer, business, or medical professional) are they?*

Again, this gets at the matter of conflict of interest, but more than that—the answer will tell you how much a part of the community, and how accountable to it, the center is.

▬ *Are the primary care-givers certified nurse-midwives? Is there a physician backup?*

77

■ *What emergency and essential life-support equipment does the center have on site? What is the emergency transfer capability and protocol?*

■ *Which hospital is the backup hospital?*

The Commission for the Accreditation of Freestanding Birth Centers is a national group spearheading the effort to enact national standards of care for freestanding birth centers and maintain high levels of quality with regard to the training and expertise of staff, the center's physical setup, and services. To find out if there is a freestanding birth center in your region *and* if it voluntarily complies with the commission's national standards, contact the National Association of Childbearing Centers, 3123 Gottschall Road, Perkiomenville, Pennsylvania 18074; telephone 1-215-234-8068.

That's the voluntary side of it. Licensing, on the other hand, is a state function, but only in those states where laws exist for such. Freestanding birth centers are subject to licensure in twenty-eight states (see page 79), under safety guidelines set up by the American Public Health Association that generally state that surgery should not be performed at the centers, labor should not be induced or hastened by Pitocin, and pain control "should depend primarily on close emotional support and adequate [childbirth] preparation."

The Home Setting

While many prospective parents are looking for home*like* and home*y* birth settings, what about the real McCoy? Is home birth a serious option? Is it safe? Ironically, the latter is a question few people think to ask about a hospital birth setting, yet the hospital is home to unnecessary surgeries, nosocomial infections, and incompetent practitioners and their often negligent practices. Home birth advocates say that home births are as safe as any other place for *normal* births, *if* there are qualified, experienced attendants and an emergency transfer system in place in case of serious complications.

Why would a woman choose to deliver at home? If she is

States Licensing
Freestanding Birth Centers

Alaska	New Hampshire
Arizona	New Mexico
California	New York
Colorado	North Carolina
Delaware	Oregon
Florida	Pennsylvania
Georgia	Rhode Island
Hawaii	Tennessee
Iowa	Texas
Kansas	Utah
Kentucky	Vermont
Maryland	Washington
Massachusetts	West Virginia
Mississippi	Wyoming

Fourteen more states and the District of Columbia are exploring the feasibility of licensure: Alabama, Arkansas, Connecticut, Illinois, Indiana, Maine, Missouri, New Jersey, Nevada, Ohio, Oklahoma, South Carolina, Virginia, and Wisconsin. And eight states have nothing: Idaho, Louisiana, Michigan, Minnesota, Montana, Nebraska, North Dakota, and South Dakota. Contact your state health department (see Appendix E) to find out about the licensure requirements your state may have.

in a remote rural setting, far from hospital or clinic, that may be her only option. A woman may also choose the home setting out of a strong desire to control the kind of childbirth she has and to give birth in a completely family-centered setting, away from intrusive hospital practices and procedures and their attendant risks. Sheila Kitzinger, a noted British childbirth educator and staunch supporter of natural childbirth and home birth, says in her book *Birth At Home* (New York: Penguin, 1979), "One of the reasons why some women want to give birth at home is that many hospitals are not good enough

. . . to provide an environment suited for a peak experience of one's life, nor for the birth of a family. But more than this, they are sometimes frankly dangerous places in which to have a baby."

People who choose home birth commonly do so amid widespread disapproval, from medical and lay sources alike. Renewed interest by women in home birth is a concept most doctors just cannot abide. They say it is dangerous, backward, and old-fashioned, and they have influence enough to have the law on their side in many cases. Undoubtedly, home birth is not for every woman or every pregnancy. If you are interested in this option, however, there is much you must do to prepare, the most important item on your agenda being the choice of birth attendant—not only the critical task of finding a competent practitioner but also the problem of finding one at all who will agree to attend a home birth. Lay midwives are your best bet because most will attend home births, as will many certified nurse-midwives; however, depending on the degree of regulation of the practice of midwifery, your state may restrict where CNMs practice. Especially in urban or even suburban areas, physicians who will attend home births are hard to find, due as much to restrictions insurance companies place on malpractice coverage as to doctors' predilection for and training in high-tech births.

There's no doubt about it: the decision to give birth at home requires a lot of planning and forethought. Not only should the prospects for the birth be as normal as can be predicted—home births are *not* for women with special health problems—but it is mandatory that you be thoroughly familiar with the process of pregnancy and birth, because you and your family or support persons are in charge of the event. Find out far in advance which childbirth method—the particular approach and preparation—you wish to use, and talk over the self-training and any medical techniques it entails with your birth practitioner. (We outline the most widely practiced methods in Chapter 6.)

The National Association of Parents and Professionals for Safe Alternatives in Childbirth (NAPSAC) has been the most visible and active organization in the movement to establish safe home births—a practice they say *should* be the norm in this country and *is* the norm throughout the world. Without home births, says the group, hospitals really have no incentive to change. To obtain more information about alternative birth services, specifically safe home births, contact the National Association of Parents and Professionals for Safe Alternatives in Childbirth, Route 1, Box 646, Marble Hill, Missouri 63764; telephone 1-314-238-2010. NAPSAC publishes a directory for people seeking a midwife, birth center, noninterventive doctor, or childbirth educator, as well as other books and tapes.

Home Births: The Dutch Experience. For some time now, the Dutch experience in obstetrics has been scrutinized by medical and public health professionals in other countries, because of the large numbers of home births and relatively low rate of medical intervention in the Netherlands. More than one-third of all children in that country (an average of 35 percent of all births) are born at home, according to a *Journal of the American Medical Association* (November 7, 1990) report. During the majority of these home deliveries (92 percent in 1987), a trained maternity nursing aide assisted the birth practitioner. In that same year, the perinatal mortality rate (defined as stillbirths and neonatal deaths within one week of birth) was 0.14 percent for those aide-assisted home births—and 0.94 percent was the national perinatal mortality rate.

Why do more than one-third of Dutch women choose home childbirth? Some of the reasons cited, says the report, are: "[The] possibility of being in control during labor; not being separated from the home environment, husband, or friends; and anxiety about (unnecessary) interventions in hospital."

Of course, important to note here is how different from ours is the system of obstetric care in the Netherlands: According to the same *Journal* article, midwives are independent practitioners who undergo three years of professional (postsecondary school) training, which qualifies them to provide care during normal pregnancy and birth; they attend some 43 percent of all deliveries. Specialist obstetricians also attend 43 percent of deliveries, and general practitioners attend 13 percent. The Dutch protocol is for midwives and general practitioners to refer women with medical or obstetric problems (according to an official list of indications) to obstetricians.

Clearly, then, the Dutch experience is in no way comparable to the components of obstetric care in the United States, but as the authors note, "[It] shows the feasibility of a system of obstetric care that combines high professional standards among those providing the care with a minimum of medical intervention as long as pregnancy and labor are normal."

CHAPTER FIVE

A Trimester-by-Trimester Guide to Obstetric Care

The First Trimester: Weeks 1 through 12

"Am I pregnant?"** This is the essential first question. After you have missed a period or you simply "feel funny"—nausea and/or inexplicable fatigue being two commonplace signs—and before you schedule an appointment to have your doctor confirm your suspicions, you can take a home pregnancy test. Of the wide variety currently on the market, all can be purchased without prescription, and all are virtually the same urine pregnancy tests performed in most doctors' offices and clinics. Some of the newest ones can detect a pregnancy as early as a few days after the missed period; with others you must wait a little longer. Although certainly not foolproof, these tests can be quite accurate if performed properly, but that's not always easy to do given the fairly complicated instructions. Recognizing the potential for confusion, the manufacturers of these products have included toll-free telephone numbers in each package insert. If you have any questions, don't hesitate to call and take advantage of a knowledgeable person—usually a registered nurse—at the other end.

The earlier the confirmation of pregnancy, the earlier you can begin proper prenatal care—for instance, avoidance of cigarettes, alcohol, drugs, and X-ray exposure—and it is especially important in the first months, when risk to the fetus is greatest. Talk to your doctor about this, and of course schedule your

How Often Should You See Your Care-giver?

Following the initial (and generally the lengthiest) office visit and calculation of the estimated delivery date, appointments typically are booked as follows (bear in mind, however, that the scheduling often depends on your medical history, whether you are considered a low- or high-risk pregnancy, and so on):

- From the first visit to 28 weeks: *every three to four weeks*
- From 28 to 32 weeks: *every three weeks*
- From 32 to 36 weeks: *every two weeks*
- From 36 weeks to delivery: *once a week*

We cannot stress enough the importance of being prepared for every visit—that is, having your research and reading done and your concerns and questions ready. Like many women, you may want to take notes. Danish women carry their own prenatal records, called "wandering journals," with them to their visits with care-givers. Why not keep a sort of medical record on yourself? A daily or weekly log of your own may be a useful tool. With it in hand, you don't have to trust your memory—"Was it before arising that morning or after eating breakfast that I felt the pain?"—and a diary can help to keep your doctor on track in those few precious (and relatively costly) minutes you have together. Use it, too, to record the results of every examination (your temperature, blood pressure, and so on), any test findings, and recommendations your doctor may make concerning prenatal care.

initial office visit as soon as you suspect or confirm that you are pregnant. We say "suspect" because even before a pregnancy test can confirm your pregnancy you may already be picking up the signals your body is giving you. Aside from a missed period, classic signs are sore and/or enlarged breasts, frequent urination, extreme fatigue, headaches, and perhaps a slightly queasy feeling.

What Happens at the Initial Doctor Visit?

Typically, this is the lengthiest, most thorough visit you will have with your obstetrician. A screening appointment, as it is sometimes called, routinely includes

- a complete medical history, including history of previous pregnancies, menstrual history, and family medical background;
- weight and blood pressure measurements;
- urine sampling to confirm pregnancy, reveal any infections, and analyze blood sugar and protein content;
- blood sampling to identify blood group, and test for venereal disease, rubella (German measles) antibodies, anemia, Rh factor (a blood incompatibility that can endanger the fetus), hepatitis, toxoplasmosis (a disease transmitted from animals, especially cats, to humans); and
- a Pap smear and internal examination to determine if the size of the uterus agrees with the estimated delivery date and to check for internal signs of pregnancy, structural abnormalities, ovarian cysts or tumors, and fibroids.

Your Due Date:
An Estimated Time of Arrival

Throughout your pregnancy you will probably hear (and think) a lot about the calculation, the concept, and the term *due date.* You'll hear your doctor refer to it, and just about everyone else you encounter talk about it—"When are you due?" "How far along are you?" "When is the blessed event?"

Who decides what it is and how? From the day of conception, or fertilization, the fetus develops for about 266 days, or 38 weeks. But because the exact date of conception can only be guessed, the progress of pregnancy usually is calculated from the first day of the woman's last menstrual period, even though she probably conceived two weeks later (depending, of course, on the length of her menstrual cycle). So doctors count 280 days, or 40 weeks.

If you believe you're pregnant, you don't have to wait for your first visit to the doctor to calculate your due date. You don't even need the specially numbered pregnancy gauge that doctors use to estimate d-day—it's not hocus-pocus or even an esoteric skill acquired only in the hallowed halls of medical schools. It's arithmetic. *If* you have a regular twenty-eight-day menstrual cycle—granted, that's an average and perhaps a big *if* in your case, but the estimated due date tables are based on it—here's what you do: Take the date of your last period, add seven days, and count three months back. For example, if your

85

last menstrual period began on July 12, count seven days ahead (with July 12 as day one)—that's July 18. Count back three months from July 18 and the date you get is April 18, which is your due date.

How important is the due date? It's hardly etched in stone, as anybody who knows anything about obstetrics can tell you, and the fact of the matter is that very few babies—experts say only one baby in twenty—arrive precisely on the date due. As an approximation, the due date has one or two weeks on either side of it that are a part of the normal time frame. Just as menstrual cycles and conception dates vary from woman to woman, so do individual pregnancies vary considerably from the average duration while still being considered normal.

Critics of modern obstetric practices talk about the "tyranny of the due date," the predilection today for many doctors to distrust their calculations *and yours* (even though many women believe they know exactly when their babies were conceived) and to rely on ultrasound to "date" the pregnancy. So dependent on technology to assess fetal maturity are some doctors that they recommend monthly ultrasounds to augment physical examinations. *Be on the lookout for such a propensity in your doctor, especially if you prefer minimal technological intervention in your pregnancy.* There is no conclusive evidence that routine ultrasonography is sound medical practice.

What Are Some of the Common Problems?

"Morning Sickness." For some women, "morning sickness," the seemingly endless nausea and, in extreme cases, vomiting, can persist all day and into the evening, becoming even more severe at mealtimes. Aside from fatigue, pregnancy sickness (as the medical literature more accurately calls it, or *hyperemesis gravidarum*, when medicos really want to get technical) is the most common complaint among women in the early weeks and months of pregnancy and represents for many women the most uncomfortable symptom of the entire pregnancy. It usually ends at completion of the first trimester or the very beginning of the second.

Ask your doctor how you can cope with these symptoms—

without drugs, which may have hazardous consequences of their own (see the discussion on Bendectin on p. 105). Although not a danger in and of itself, pregnancy sickness, if it is severe and of long duration, may result in substantial weight loss. Talk to your doctor about any pregnancy sickness you're having and any weight loss you're experiencing. Ask at what point weight loss becomes severe enough to require hospitalization and/or intravenous feeding. No doubt you will want to avoid this; therefore, discuss what preventive measures you can take so that the situation doesn't take such a turn.

Bleeding or Spotting. Bleeding during the first trimester is common, and in some instances occasional bleeding (spotting) can continue throughout the pregnancy without danger. At the same time, bleeding is a warning sign that you should bring to the attention of your doctor—because early in pregnancy it *may be* an indication of a serious problem such as a threatened miscarriage or an ectopic pregnancy (see pp. 88–91). Your doctor can distinguish between minor spotting and symptoms of more serious problems, which is why it is imperative that you notify her as soon as any spotting or bleeding occurs.

Heartburn and Constipation. Considered more likely to occur during the final months, heartburn is not uncommon in the early stages. And as with constipation, another common complaint during pregnancy, you need to talk to your doctor about nondrug treatments. Medications of any kind, even over-the-counter concoctions, should be carefully screened. Talk to your doctor about nonprescription remedies but also corroborate her recommendations with your pharmacist. (Or if you really want to get the best from a team approach to medical care, have your primary care-giver—your doctor—call the drug expert, your pharmacist, and let them powwow over the best course. Then hear their recommendations.)

What Complications May Arise?

The majority of pregnancies progress normally and uneventfully through the first trimester. This is not to say that complications don't arise; they do—spontaneously, in a healthy woman with no obvious risk factors, or as a result of known risk factors such as poor nutrition, smoking, alcohol consumption, high blood pressure, and family history of disease.

Miscarriage. What most of us call miscarriage the medical world calls spontaneous abortion. Between 15 and 20 percent of clinically recognized pregnancies abort spontaneously, often completely unnoticed by the woman. Miscarriages most often occur between weeks 6 and 10, according to many experts.

Why do miscarriages occur? The leading causes are fetal abnormality, maternal hormonal imbalance, and anatomical defects of the uterus. Other factors associated with increased risk of miscarriage include drug and alcohol use, genetic defects, and exposure to environmental toxins. *It is generally acknowledged that pregnant women whose mothers took the synthetic hormone DES (diethylstilbestrol) during their pregnancy have increased risk of miscarriage. If this is true of you, be sure to tell your doctor.* In individual cases, though, the exact cause often remains unknown.

How will you know if a miscarriage is impending? Slight bleeding or spotting, although not always indicative of a threatened miscarriage, nevertheless may signal one. Other signs include severe abdominal pain, severe cramps, dizziness, and even blurred or double vision. But if you are experiencing nothing other than bleeding or spotting, be aware that some miscarriages are completely painless. *If you experience any vaginal bleeding in pregnancy, you should consult your doctor.*

Ask when she considers the bleeding substantial or otherwise worrisome enough to merit further examination, perhaps even testing to find the reason. A three-step evaluation is a typical avenue for doctors to take: internal pelvic examination to check the condition of the uterus and cervix; blood test to determine the health of the pregnancy by measuring the level of human chorionic gonadotropin (HCG), a hormone secreted by the placenta; and ultrasonography. If your doctor feels that the bleeding is caused by an impending miscarriage, ask what you can do to stop the bleeding and cramping and help the pregnancy proceed to full term. In other words, is there anything you can do to *prevent* a miscarriage? Does your doctor recommend bed rest, or cessation of any particular activities such as sexual intercourse? What about exercise? Should you continue working? When does your doctor believe hospitalization is necessary? Why and for how long?

If it turns out that you *are* miscarrying: What must the doctor do? When is a D&C (dilation and curettage) necessary? How long does it take to recover from a miscarriage and resume normal activities? How soon can you try to get pregnant again? And what are your chances of having another miscarriage? If this is not your first miscarriage, ask about further testing by a geneticist or infertility specialist. The answers to the above questions have a great deal to do with your current and past medical history. Be sure your doctor is up to date on your past experiences.

You and your doctor need to look at it from all angles—the physical process of miscarriage, and the physical *and* emotional recovery. Ask your doctor to recommend any local support groups that specialize in helping women and couples cope with the emotional aftermath of miscarriage. (We list national groups in Appendix I.) Along with community centers, local women's groups, and churches and synagogues in your area, you might call the local hospitals, who may also have begun organizing pregnancy-loss support groups.

Finding Out What Caused Your Miscarriage

Experts believe that as many as one in three pregnancies fails, and women who have miscarried once stand a greater chance of repeating the experience unless the problem is diagnosed and treated. Stefan Semchyshyn, M.D., writing in his book *How to Prevent Miscarriage and Other Crises of Pregnancy* (New York: Collier Books, 1990), debunks the myth that miscarriage is nature's way of terminating a defective fetus and says the problem in at least one-third of all miscarriage cases is a maternal medical problem. Semchyshyn, a maternal and fetal medicine specialist and leading authority on high-risk pregnancy, dismisses what he calls the "standard medical practice"of waiting for two, three, or more miscarriages before investigating more closely. He urges women to work with their physicians after the *first loss* or, of course, before, to prevent the tragedy of subsequent miscarriages or even a first one.

Some of the conditions Semchyshyn and others associate with miscarriage include

- a weakened cervix, which some women are born with, although an abortion or a previous miscarriage can also weaken the cervix;
- chromosomal abnormality;
- maternal age—thirty-five or older;
- maternal illness—such as sexually transmitted diseases, hypertension, or diabetes;
- obesity;
- hormonal insufficiency, resulting in an inadequate production of progesterone;
- history of infertility, previous miscarriage, or premature birth; and
- retroverted, or backward-tilted, uterus, which affects about 30 percent of all women.

Ectopic, or Tubal, Pregnancy. A pregnancy is ectopic when the fertilized egg does not complete its descent but begins to develop outside the uterus, usually in one of the fallopian tubes— hence the term *tubal pregnancy.* Occasionally, the fertilized egg may start to grow in the mother's abdominal cavity or on the ovary. Far less common than miscarriages, ectopic pregnancy occurs in about 1.5 percent of all pregnancies, according to the Centers for Disease Control (*Morbidity and Mortality Weekly Report,* December 1988), and this figure represents a tripling of the rate since 1970.

How do you know if your pregnancy is ectopic? What are the symptoms? The classic signs are cramps and spotting early in the pregnancy, sometimes even before the woman is aware that she is pregnant, and, subsequently, more bleeding and severe lower abdominal pain. As already noted, bleeding and pain may also signal impending miscarriage, among other things, so be sure to call your doctor or seek other medical advice *whenever you experience bleeding.*

Ectopic pregnancy, called "one of the true obstetric emergencies" in an article in *The Female Patient* (October 1989), always results in the loss of the fetus and is now one of the leading causes of maternal death in this country, according to the Centers for Disease Control. So every woman should be alert to the possibility of ectopic pregnancy. Know the symptoms, and go over them with your doctor no later than the screening appointment.

How can you prevent or avoid an ectopic pregnancy? You can't, but you should know the risk factors and talk to your doctor about their pertinence to your individual case *way ahead of becoming pregnant.* In fact, a particularly thorough medical history in the prepregnancy planning stage should raise the red flags associated with increased risk—a history of pelvic inflammatory disease, history of endometriosis, prior tubal surgery, history of infertility, use of IUDs for contraception, and previous ectopic pregnancy. Cigarette smoking has also emerged in new studies as a potential risk factor (*American Journal of Public Health*, September 1989).

It is crucial to diagnose an ectopic pregnancy before the tube ruptures. If you specifically are at risk and have any of the symptoms of an ectopic pregnancy, ask your doctor what diagnostic and treatment options you have. Does he first perform a blood test to measure levels of HCG? (Most do.) Is there any drug treatment available? What about imaging technology such as ultrasonography to locate the pregnancy? Or laparoscopy? (Laparoscopy is a visual examination of the lower abdomen with a telescopic instrument inserted through a small incision.)

Once an ectopic pregnancy is confirmed, surgical removal of the pregnancy must be performed immediately, prior to rupture. At this point, the questions for your doctor are these: "What is your experience in such surgery?" "How many times have you performed the delicate microsurgery mandatory to saving the fallopian tube?" However, be aware that once the tube has burst, you may have severe hemorrhage, and in this case the general medical opinion is: Protecting the tube is a low priority because there is no time for delicate surgical techniques. Still, you want to know what your doctor's skills and expertise are, and if they're not so great, insist on a competent, experienced surgeon.

Should You Be Tested for the Presence of AIDS Antibodies?

An increasing number of doctors are recommending that pregnant women undergo HIV (human immunodeficiency virus) antibody testing. HIV is the virus that causes acquired immune deficiency syndrome (AIDS), and it is capable of crossing the placenta and infecting the developing fetus. Because not everyone with the virus has developed AIDS, a pregnant woman can feel perfectly well but still have passed on the virus to the fetus. Women at high risk are

- intravenous drug users;
- women whose sexual partners are intravenous drug users or bisexual;
- prostitutes or women who have had sexual partners with AIDS or whose background may not be known to them; and
- women who have had blood transfusions before 1985 (before screening of donated blood by the AIDS antibody test).

Talk to your doctor.

What Tests Will Your Doctor Recommend?

Tests present a dilemma for the pregnant woman. She doesn't want to neglect to have a critical test, *if* it is indeed critical and *if* indeed the results will enable her and her doctor to work together to arrive at an informed decision about her health and her baby's. Then there is the dilemma, the very real problem, of interventionism in pregnancy without sound medical basis—over- and unnecessary testing being only one but a principal aspect of it. Our best advice here, as elsewhere, is that you get complete information about the purposes and also the results of all tests.

Prenatal tests can be invaluable in the early detection of fetal neural tube defects such as spina bifida (some of the vertebrae fail to close, thereby exposing the spinal cord) and anencephaly (incomplete development of the brain). About one in every one thousand infants born in the United States is born with a neural tube defect, and more than 90 percent of these cases of fetal defects occur in families who have no familial history of such (*Female Patient*, October 1989).

How to Prevent Testitis

Here is a quick checklist of questions to ask your doctor when a test is recommended:

- "How much will the test cost?"
- "What preparation is necessary?"
- "How long before the test results are ready?"
- "What will you be looking for in the results of these tests?" "What do you hope to learn from the test and how accurate is it?" The first is a key question because it requires your doctor to let you in on the process, diagnosis, and prognosis, and to justify the need for further testing. As far as the latter is concerned, your doctor should be discussing the test's false-positive and false-negative rates and what they may mean for retesting and so on.
- "Will the procedure be painful and is it dangerous?" Don't hesitate to ask this question because a test may cause more pain (or may lead to complications more dangerous) than the benefit to be derived from the test results. This is usually not the case, but in this era of high technology with little oversight of its safety and benefit, a smart consumer questions her doctor about the efficacy of the tests he recommends.
- "Do the potential benefits of the tests outweigh the tests' risks?" The tests themselves might be dangerous or cause serious problems. Have your doctor give you a rundown of the possibilities.
- "Is this the most appropriate test?" Tests are big money for doctors and facilities. Today any number of tests are used to diagnose or rule out a condition. Because of this, many doctors have fallen victim to "testitis"—they use all the tests available instead of the most comprehensive one. Watch out for the doctor who wants to move you up the test ladder. Ask why he is not recommending the most comprehensive one *first*. Remember, one comprehensive test may be much cheaper than three lesser ones.
- "What will happen if I don't have this procedure done?" This is a question you must ask. It may be the single most important query anyone could pose at any and every level of dealings with the medical system, and it should be asked every time a procedure is recommended. What could you possibly lose by asking? And you could gain a great deal.

There are advantages to knowing beforehand if your baby has health problems, but what if the test that made such a pronouncement is unreliable? Or what if the problem is incurable? Approximately 250 birth defects can be diagnosed in the unborn fetus, but that is far more than can be treated or cured.

Personal decisions, too, must be made. Do you risk miscarriage (a potential complication of both amniocentesis and chorionic villus sampling) of a healthy fetus because the prospect of delivering a baby with birth defects is unacceptable to you? Should the test results indicate a problem, is elective termination of pregnancy—abortion—acceptable to you? If not, do you agree to the test "just to know"?

These are just a few of the dilemmas that prenatal tests and their results can create. If you already know that you are the carrier of a genetic defect, then the decision to undergo prenatal tests is probably a fairly easy one—and perhaps it is also if you're over age thirty-five and having your first baby. Ordered routinely for increasing numbers of women, however, prenatal tests necessitate a lot of questions and discussions of relative risks and benefits.

Chorionic Villus Sampling. Depending on your age and perhaps your past obstetric history, between week 8 and week 12 your doctor may order chorionic villus sampling (CVS)—one of the newest tests available to help determine whether your baby has a chromosomal abnormality such as Down syndrome. Current medical wisdom holds that a woman over age thirty-five is at higher risk of conceiving such a child. Aside from maternal age, two other factors may predispose a woman to CVS: if she (or her partner) has a family history of genetic disorders, or if she has a previous child with a birth defect. A newer test and considered an alternative to the more well known amniocentesis, CVS has the advantage that it can be performed earlier than amniocentesis—usually in the first trimester—and results can be determined earlier, too: usually less than a week to reveal Down syndrome and about two weeks for a more thorough analysis. Unlike amniocentesis, CVS offers the woman the option of a safer first-trimester abortion, should early test results indicate a problem and she decides to terminate the pregnancy. It can also allow more time for follow-up testing.

But when risk of miscarriage and other complications is taken into account, the picture is less than perfect, say critics. Complications noted, but for which there are no measurements or numbers, are intrauterine growth retardation; prematurity, or early labor; and infection. For the past few years, the jury on CVS has been rather neatly divided into two factions: those who say that the precedure carries nearly the same risk of miscarriage as does amniocentesis (and the distinct advantage of earlier testing), and those who say the risk is at least twice that of amniocentesis (the American College of Obstetricians and Gynecologists says between 0.5 and 1 percent). Very early reports on the rate of fetal loss with CVS were even higher, and for some time CVS was considered experimental by the American College of Obstetricians and Gynecologists. It no longer is (*when* performed by properly trained physicians).

The National Institutes of Health, National Institute of Child Health and Human Development, in a large, multicenter study, conducted some of the newest and most significant research comparing the safety of CVS with that of amniocentesis. Writing in the *New England Journal of Medicine* (March 9, 1989), investigators concluded that CVS "is a safe and effective technique for the early prenatal diagnosis of [chromosome] abnormalities, but that it probably entails a slightly higher risk of procedure failure and of fetal loss than does amniocentesis." Another national study, this one Canadian and of similar scope and size as the American, compared CVS and amniocentesis in thousands of pregnancies, and arrived at the same conclusion—that CVS is probably slightly riskier than amniocentesis (*Lancet,* January 7, 1989).

Both the American and the Canadian studies employed *transcervical* chorionic villus sampling, in which, with the woman in the lithotomy position, a thin tube is passed into the vagina and through the cervix. (As with amniocentesis, ultrasound is necessary to locate the appropriate site for sampling.) A very small sample of tissue is taken from the chorionic villi, finger-shaped projections of the fetal sac that later will develop into the placenta. From this sample, chromosome abnormalities can be detected. An alternative to the transcervical route is *transabdominal* CVS. In this, the woman is in the more comfortable supine position, and with ultrasound guidance a needle is inserted through the abdominal wall and the sample obtained. Until recently, transcervical CVS was the only technique in use in this country, but the transabdominal approach has been rapidly gaining popularity, primarily because it minimizes the possibility of intrauterine infection.

According to a Baylor College of Medicine study reported in the *American Journal of Obstetrics and Gynecology* (November 1989), in varying degrees other complications are about the same: spotting and bleeding (relatively common following transcervical CVS, and less frequent in transabdominal); mild cramping (occasional in transcervical, and common but short-lived in transabdominal); and fetal loss (risk about the same for both techniques).

Supporters of the transabdominal approach say that a woman whose pregnancy is too advanced for safe transcervical CVS—for example, a pregnancy somewhere between weeks 12 and 14, which would require a wait even to have an amniocentesis—should be able to choose transabdominal CVS, "a reliable alternative approach" (*Bailliere's Clinical Obstetrics and Gynecology*, September 1987).

All well and good, except that few doctors and technicians have the same level of expertise and experience in both methods, if they have any expertise and experience at all in transabdominal CVS, the less popular method. And fewer hospitals around the nation offer chorionic villus sampling than offer amniocentesis, simply because CVS is the newer technique.

────── *Other First-Trimester Tests and Measurements*

After your first visit, the screening appointment, your subsequent prenatal visits fall into a pattern, and you can expect the same tests every time you see the doctor, but don't take even the routine tests lying down. Question, question, question—that's the best way to stay in control of your health and pregnancy and to maximize the time spent with your doctor.

Incidence of Genetic Disorders

Down syndrome

Maternal Age	Occurrence in Live Births
35	1 in 378
40	1 in 106
45	1 in 30

All chromosome diseases

Maternal Age	Occurrence in Live Births
20	1 in 526
35	1 in 192
40	1 in 66
45	1 in 21

All ages (15–44)

Disorder	Occurrence in Live Births
Beta thalassemia	1 in 2,500 to 1 in 800
Cystic fibrosis	1 in 2,500
Down syndrome	1 in 800
Hemophilia	1 in 2,500 (males)
Huntington's disease	1 in 15,000
Klinefelter syndrome	1 in 800 (males)
Sickle-cell anemia	1 in 625
Tay-Sachs disease	1 in 3,600

Source: American College of Obstetricians and Gynecologists.

● *Weight and Blood Pressure Measurements.* Ask your doctor "What is considered normal?" and "How am I doing relative to 'normal'?" Your doctor will probably tell you that a blood pressure slightly above your normal prepregnant level is nothing to worry about—ask how high it must be before it *is* something to worry about. And, if you wish, monitor your own blood pressure at home, taking measurements at varying times of the day so as to get a truer picture. ("White-coat hypertension"

97

Some Questions to Ask

Along with your questions concerning the purpose, necessity, and risks and benefits of any prenatal test, and in this case chorionic villus sampling, be prepared to ask about the hospital's or lab's experience, and the expertise of the doctors and other staff. There has long been talk of "learning curves," a concept especially critical with procedures so relatively new that many doctors did not train for them in medical school. And given the routine application of amniocentesis and the growing popularity of CVS, you have to wonder if everyone performing the test knows what he is doing. Are their skills up to par? Study after study has shown that various factors have impact on expertise: "operator" (doctor) experience; technician experience; and lab quality.

Also keep in mind that with experience comes economy, in the sense that the doctor who is expert in the procedure makes fewer "passes" to obtain an amount of fluid adequate for sampling—and this means that you will spend less time and have less discomfort undergoing the test.

Find out:

● Which medical facility or hospital is best for the particular test? Which doctor? Ask how frequent the procedure is performed and the complication rates.

● What is their experience? How many such tests have they performed? How long have they been doing these procedures?

● What is the false-positive rate (meaning that the test results indicate a birth defect when there actually is none) for the test at that facility? False-negative rate (meaning that the test results indicate no birth defect when there actually is one)?

● What are the qualifications of the lab analyzing the sample? What is its typical turnaround time for the test—in other words, how long before you and your doctor know the results?

● What is the lab's retest rate? Occasionally, test results are botched at the lab. Aside from the risks and discomfort associated with another test, there is further delay.

is a very real phenomenon, described at great length in many medical journals and clearly something your doctor should know about. It refers to the finding that blood pressure measurements taken at the doctor's office may not be truly representative of the person's average daily pressure. Not only is "bp" a constantly changing variable, but it is a known fact that many people suffer from an above-normal rise in blood pressure provoked by the anxiety associated with a visit to the doctor.)

- *Weight.* The whole question of what weight is ideal throughout the different stages of pregnancy is controversial, so you should spend a lot of time discussing this with your doctor and tailoring the recommended weights (see below) to your unique situation—your build, your prepregnancy weight, and your level of activity and exercise. Here's a sample of how your doctor might be interpreting the latest medical thinking on approximately how much weight should be gained and when (based on an average weight gain of 25 pounds as ideal):

During the first 2½ to 3 months: *2 to 3 pounds*
At 20 weeks: *a total gain of about 8 pounds*
At 30 weeks: *a total gain of about 15 pounds*
At 40 weeks: *a total gain of about 25 pounds*

- *Urinalysis.* Must you bring in a urine specimen each time you visit the doctor? Collected when? Refrigerated? Can you provide one on the spot? Urine test results may be inaccurate if the specimen is collected at the wrong time, stored improperly, or contaminated somehow. David S. Sobel, M.D., and Tom Ferguson, M.D., in *The People's Book of Medical Tests* (New York: Summit Books, 1985), differentiate among four types of urine specimens: random specimen; first-morning specimen; second-voided specimen; and timed specimen. Talk to your doctor about this.

- *Examination for Edema.* Your ankles, fingers, and legs will be checked for swelling due to fluid in the tissues. Ask your doctor how much swelling is considered normal and what you can do to minimize it and prevent it from worsening. (Make sure the recommended therapies do not involve drugs, such as diuretics, now considered risky during pregnancy.)

- *Examination of Your Abdomen.* Although you probably will not be able to feel the top of your womb above your pubic bone until sometime around or after week 12, at each visit your doctor will check the size and growth of the uterus. She is looking for a uterus growing faster than expected—perhaps indicating a large baby or multiple birth—or growing slower than expected, perhaps due to problems in fetal growth.

99

——— *A Word About Self-Care*

Why not take the reins of control—in this case, a sphygmomanometer, or blood pressure gauge; a dipstick, for urine testing; a tape measure, for measuring your uterus; and a bathroom scale, for comparing your home assessment with the physician's assessment of your weight—and evaluate and record your own blood pressure, uterine size, and so on? Self-care is involving and empowering, and what better way to be an equal partner with your physician in your own medical care?

——— *Weight Gain:*
How Much Is Too Much?
(Or Even Too Little?)

For years the question has been bandied about among doctors, dietitians, pregnant women, and mothers and mothers-in-law, and the answers have fluctuated as wildly as fashions. Vogue for a while was the philosophy that to gain an ounce over 15 or 16 pounds was unhealthy for the baby and certainly impractical for the woman, who would have too much weight to lose after the birth. True, more than merely a fashion statement, the suggested poundage was based on the theory that excessive weight gain caused toxemia, a condition characterized by increased blood pressure, inordinate swelling, and protein in the urine. That theory has since been discarded—probably because research found the contrary to be true: good nutrition can prevent toxemia, and malnutrition (especially lack of protein) is partly responsible for it.

Trendy at one time, along with restricted caloric intake, was restricted salt intake. Many pregnant women even were given diuretics, or "water pills," which eliminate fluids from the body. For the most part, that recommendation has fallen by the wayside, as studies show that salt is essential to pregnant women and growing babies. However, although the American College of Obstetricians and Gynecologists (ACOG) advises against routine sodium restriction (unless the woman has a preexisting condition that requires a low-salt diet), some

100

Before Your First Trimester Is Over

● Discuss with your doctor where you want to deliver your baby. (See Chapter 4 for information on various birth settings, their pros and cons, and the questions to ask about each during the decision-making process.) You may still be adjusting to the idea of being pregnant and thinking it awfully early to be planning so far down the road, but it isn't. You can always change your mind.

● Get started on a birth plan (see p. 65 and Appendix F), especially if you have decided on the hospital as your birth setting. Now is the time to lay the groundwork for a safe and satisfying birth experience.

● Talk turkey—cold turkey, that is, if you are a smoker. Ask your physician to help. Who knows until you ask? Also get your doctor's views on caffeine and alcohol consumption.

● Ask your doctor what you can take for a headache, stomachache, indigestion, hay fever and allergy symptoms, and so on—in short, all the little annoyances about which most of us never think twice before self-doctoring with an over-the-counter remedy.

● Talk money! Find out what your doctor charges for the entire maternity care package—from prenatal office visits through delivery and postpartum care. Then contact your company benefits manager (if you work) or your insurance company (if you are otherwise insured) to see what is covered and not covered. If you plan to pay entirely out of your own pocket, now is the time to negotiate the doctor's fee and set up a payment schedule.

● Enroll in early pregnancy classes, a new concept in parent education programs and usually offered during the first and second trimesters, if you and your partner feel you want help dealing with the early and ongoing physical and emotional changes of pregnancy. Check with your local Y or other community center.

● Find a partner. If the baby's father is not the one who will be acting as advocate, partner, and/or coach throughout your pregnancy and childbirth, find someone who will! Whomever you choose should start *now*, if possible—and accompany you as you test the waters with your chosen birth attendant, navigate through prenatal office visits, and set sail with early childbirth preparation classes. We cannot overemphasize the importance of having such a person with you as you go through your pregnancy and childbirth experience.

doctors continue to place pregnant women on low-salt diets and prescribe diuretics.

As you can see, answers to the question of "How much?" or "How little?" are subject to the whims of medical science and folk wisdom, which is precisely why you need to tread cautiously. The current trend is for doctors to specify a 24- to 28-pound weight gain (ACOG's 1988 "Guidelines for Perinatal Care" advise 22 to 27, but indicate that higher is okay, too). This is an average, doctors say, but as more than one critic has pointed out, too often the average becomes the ideal. Not exactly arbitrary, the figures result from a formula of how much "everything" weighs: Of the 24 to 28 pounds, the baby accounts for 10.5 pounds—7.5 for the fetus, 1 for the placenta, and 2 for the amniotic fluid. The remaining pounds belong to the mother—4 to 6 for fat and nutrient stores, 5 to 7 for increases in blood and fluid volume, 2.5 for the uterus, and 2 for breast enlargement [*The Columbia University College of Physicians and Surgeons Complete Guide to Pregnancy* (New York: Crown, 1988)]. The recommended weight gain works out to about 1 pound per week after the first trimester, or several hundred extra calories a day over prepregnancy levels.

So eat as much as you want, salt your food to taste, and gain at least 24 pounds—that's the general medical advice of the day, but it is not very helpful with specifics: What are adequate amounts of protein and essential vitamins and minerals? What about vitamin and mineral supplementation? ("Moderate use" is usually advised here, but is that enough? And how much is too much?) And what problems does a vegetarian diet (or some such variation) pose? Much of the criticism aimed at doctors also revolves around the negative approach many take in nutritional counseling: "So, Ms. X, you've gained eight pounds this month—that's too much. You've got to cut down."

More than family practitioners, obstetricians are the major culprits here. Their training, as we emphasize throughout this book, points them to technological interventions—tests, drugs, surgery—when there are problems in pregnancy, and not to preventive measures such as good nutrition. Nutrition is largely ignored in the medical curriculum, so doctors have next to nothing in the way of nutritional training. Is it any wonder, then, that "Eat a balanced diet" is about as close as some doctors come to dietary counseling?

Clearly, the key is that you become your own nutritionist, and be prepared to seek the counseling of a bona fide nutritionist, if you feel you need help beyond your own or your doctor's resources. And, perhaps more here than in any other area of prenatal care, it is important to have a take-charge attitude, because what you eat (and don't eat) has a direct effect on your baby's health, not to mention your health and even the type of labor and delivery you will have. As scant on specific (or practical) articles on prenatal nutrition as the medical literature is, the popular press fortunately is a veritable cornucopia of advice, ranging from the traditional "four basic food groups" school of thought to alternative approaches.

Exercise

The days when a pregnant woman was told to do no exercise more strenuous than walking are behind us, but the dust is still settling in the medical world after years of skirmishes over *exactly* what level of maternal activity interferes with fetal development. For some years now, research findings have ricocheted like tennis balls around the pages of medical and popular literature. So you're likely to read or hear several different, sometimes contradictory viewpoints:

- "Strenuous exercise during pregnancy may result in a low-birth-weight baby."

- "Babies born to women who exercise are usually full term with normal birth weights and do not show any significant incidences of low Apgar scores [a scoring method given twice in the minutes following delivery to quickly evaluate the condition of the infant at birth, specifically muscle tone, heart rate, respiratory effort, reflex irritability, and color]."

- "Strenuous exercise during pregnancy may result in certain prenatal complications such as early pregnancy loss, decreased maternal weight gain, impaired placental and fetal growth, and preterm labor."

103

- "During early pregnancy, physically fit women can continue to perform aerobic exercise at intensities between 50 and 85 percent of maximum, without significantly increasing their risk of miscarriage."

With all these voices and your own desires to take into account, what do you do? Realize, of course, that the best time to begin an exercise program is before becoming pregnant, and that it is not wise to begin a vigorous exercise program during pregnancy if you have not done so before.

Talk over with your doctor the sorts of activities you did before and wish to continue, and ask what general guidelines he advises. There's a good chance your doctor cleaves to the current medical dicta, so familiarize yourself with the American College of Obstetricians and Gynecologists guidelines:

─────── *During Pregnancy*

1. Maternal heart rate should not exceed 140 beats per minute.
2. Strenuous activities should not exceed fifteen minutes in duration.
3. No exercise should be performed while lying on your back after the fourth month of pregnancy is completed.
4. Exercises that employ the Valsalva maneuver (strong bearing down) should be avoided.
5. Caloric intake should be adequate to meet the extra energy needs of pregnancy and exercise.
6. Maternal core temperature should not exceed 99.6° F (38° C).

More generally speaking, ACOG recommends that pregnant women exercise regularly, at least three times a week, but discourages strenuous exercise and competitive games. Also:

- Avoid bouncy, jerky, or twisting movements, rapid changes in direction and speed, and deep, unsupported stretching.
- Exercise on a wood or carpeted floor or an exercise pad.
- Avoid exercise in hot, humid weather or when you have a fever.
- Begin exercise with a five-minute warm-up and follow with a cool-down of similar duration.

- Measure heart rate at peak activity level.
- Rise gradually from the floor and continue some form of leg activity for a while.
- Take liquids before and after exercise (or even during, if necessary).
- Stop activity and contact your care-giver if any unusual symptoms appear: sudden or severe chest pain or headache; irregular or rapid heartbeat; uterine contractions; vaginal bleeding; fainting, dizziness, confusion; and so on.

If exercise intensity is the issue, the formulas or rules hardly apply equally to everyone. For the older, more sedentary woman, for instance, a heart rate of 140 is probably way too high, but maybe not for the long-distance runner, who can probably tolerate a more intense workout. So, again, tailor your discussions to your own level of physical fitness and your own unique circumstances—hypertension or a history of miscarriages or premature labor, for example, usually make vigorous activity during pregnancy undesirable.

Before we move on to the second trimester, two other topics of note should be mentioned: the question of medications during pregnancy, and X rays.

- *Medications During Pregnancy.* The thalidomide tragedy of the 1960s and the more recent controversy over the popular antinausea drug Bendectin bring into sharp focus the undeniable fact that some medications routinely prescribed are harmful when taken during pregnancy. The fact that the Food and Drug Administration has approved a drug for use does not necessarily guarantee that the drug is safe for use.

In the case of Bendectin, for more than twenty years the drug was used by tens of millions of women worldwide for the treatment of "morning sickness," a common discomfort of early pregnancy. Amid the rampant prescribing and medical acceptance of the drug's safety, reports began to circulate alleging Bendectin's link to birth defects. There were even accusations of a cover-up on the part of the drug manufacturer and the Food and Drug Administration, but it wasn't until some years later, in 1983, that Bendectin was taken off the market.

Presumably, the doctor who prescribes any medication for

105

the pregnant woman considers the drug absolutely essential or he wouldn't write that "scrip," right? Well, maybe. But often the doctor does not really know anything about the drug; he just knows that "X is what I always give women to reduce swelling" or "Y will remedy your constipation" or "Z is the best thing on the market for sleeplessness." In a survey conducted by the journal *Drug Topics*, 21 percent of retail pharmacists reported catching ten or more medication errors each week in physician prescribing, including physician miscalculation of dosage and out-and-out wrong selection of drug, as well as errors involving inaccurate or incomplete directions for taking the drug—the most frequent kind of error in this survey. These figures are not meant as scare tactics, just reminders to work *with* your practitioner in any and all medical decisions made at this time.

The American Academy of Pediatrics says that no drug has been proved safe for the unborn child, so proceed with caution. Make your doctor specify the urgent medical need for every medication prescribed during pregnancy, but realize, too, that you share in that responsibility. Your goal should be to avoid chemical substances, if at all possible, and if that presents a real problem or there is a real medical necessity, obtain all the information you can about the drug. You can consult the *Physicians' Desk Reference*, which is a compilation of drug industry package inserts and probably the primary resource your doctor uses, but there are other, perhaps less biased publications for the information. Here are a few (with the publisher listed in parentheses): *Advice for the Patient: Drug Information in Lay Language* (United States Pharmacopoeial Convention, 1990); *Springhouse Drug Reference* (Springhouse Corporation, 1988); and *The Essential Guide to Prescription Drugs* (Harper & Row, 1988).

Then discuss with your practitioner whether the symptom you're suffering (nausea, headache, runny nose, or whatever) or the problem you're having is preferable to the side effects and possible damage to the baby caused by the remedy.

- *X Rays During Pregnancy.* What's the quibble, you ask, when everyone knows that X rays should be avoided whenever possible during pregnancy? Even with this dictum, it doesn't do to become complacent because there may come a time during your pregnancy when your doctor believes one is necessary.

It certainly is not unheard of for a doctor to order an X ray to measure the dimensions and capacity of the pelvis to determine if it is large enough to allow a vaginal birth, in the event of a breech presentation, for example. Generally performed late in the pregnancy, diagnostic pelvimetry, as it's called, is not without risk to the fetus. In their book *X-rays: Health Effects of Common Exams* (San Francisco: Sierra Club Books, 1985), John W. Gofman, M.D., Ph.D., and Egan O'Connor detail and formularize this risk: "A fetus receives a whole-body dose of 0.75 rad during her mother's pelvimetry exam. What will be the child's resulting risk of getting a radiation-induced cancer sometime during her lifetime? . . . 22,504 per million, or one chance in 44."

To kick off discussion—because before you consent to have such an X ray, you should *be convinced* of the overriding necessity of it—show this statistic to your doctor if and when such a test is recommended, and also tell her that these authors are not triflers: Gofman, a physician and doctor of nuclear/physical chemistry, and professor emeritus at the University of California at Berkeley, discovered Uranium-233 while in graduate school, worked for the Manhattan Project in the 1940s, and has been honored for his extensive work on cancer, chromosomes, radiation, and human health.

It is unlikely that while pregnant you will be asked to have an X ray, and in any case the order of business should be for the doctor—chiropractor, family practitioner, or whatever—to ask you the right question right off, before ordering, much less performing, an X ray examination: "Are you pregnant?"

The Second Trimester: Weeks 13 through 26

What Tests Will Your Doctor Recommend?

Alpha Fetoprotein Screening. Alpha fetoprotein (AFP) is a protein produced by the fetus early in uterine life and present in the amniotic fluid and in smaller amounts in the mother's bloodstream. (The term *maternal serum alpha fetoprotein*, often shortened to MSAFP, is synonymous with our use of AFP.) A certain level of AFP in the mother's blood is considered normal, but unusual levels (either high or low) suggest potential problems. Abnormally high levels are associated with a variety of birth defects, especially neural tube defects such as spina bifida, in which part of the spinal column is exposed through an opening, and anencephaly, in which part of the skull is missing and the brain improperly formed. Elevated levels are also often present in women carrying twins and when the fetus has died in utero. Because the amount of AFP varies during pregnancy, an elevated reading may also be due to a miscalculation of gestational age, or length of pregnancy. An abnormally low level of AFP may indicate Down syndrome.

All that is needed for the screening, usually done between 15 and 20 weeks into the pregnancy, is a blood sample from the mother. And the results are typically ready in three to five days, although it may take up to a week or two. The major benefits of AFP screening? It involves a relatively simple blood test, taken at your doctor's office, and provides an opportunity to find out about your baby's health before it is born. So where's the need for caution? You would be wise to keep in mind that the blood test is not a truly diagnostic test, but a screening; it indicates those women who are *most likely* to be carrying affected fetuses. And AFP screening is not foolproof. Spina bifidas may go undetected. Women with high levels of AFP have been found to be carrying healthy babies, and in this case in order to confirm a specific diagnosis, further testing must be done. Such a situation is not uncommon: The first blood test and even a follow-up blood test show an elevated AFP level, so an ultrasound is done to confirm the gestational date, to determine whether the pregnant woman is carrying twins and to reveal any defects that may exist. If no neural tube defect is seen, the stage of pregnancy is accurate, and the woman is not carrying twins, amniocentesis is done to measure the AFP level in the amniotic fluid.

Most women with high AFP levels on the first and even the second blood test will turn out to be carrying normal, healthy fetuses (or perhaps twins), a fact that will be determined by ultrasound and/or amniocentesis. Norra Tannenhaus, in her book *Preconceptions*, reports: "Of every 1,000 women who take the test, perhaps 50 will have suspiciously high levels of AFP. But of those 50, only two will probably have a child with a neural tube defect. Of the remaining 48, some will test normal on a second try; most will be found to have inaccurately dated their pregnancies; still others will be found to have multiple babies. Some will have babies with other forms of defects, and some will have normal babies for whom no reason for elevated AFP levels can be found."

So discuss this with your doctor and weigh your options. Just remember that routine AFP screening subjects *many* women to a series of tests. True, every diagnostic test along the way increases the chances and accuracy with which the relatively few cases of neural tube effects are diagnosed. Talk to your doctor about the screening's value in your own circumstances. Know the facts: "[The] test *does* have limitations. It cannot detect all birth defects. It will yield some false-positive results in which no abnormalities are found. It can also produce false-negative results, which means an abnormality is present in the fetus, but is not detected by the test" (*Journal of Pediatric Healthcare*, May/June 1989).

Amniocentesis. First pioneered in the 1950s, amniocentesis involves the sampling and examination of fetal cells floating in amniotic fluid. With the help of ultrasound to locate the fetus and placenta, a needle is inserted through the woman's abdomen and into the uterus. A small amount of the fluid surrounding the baby is removed. Sometimes a local anesthetic is used, sometimes not, and on infrequent occasions the doctor may have to make another "pass" to get enough amniotic fluid.

The test is most often used to detect Down syndrome, but it can also detect other chromosome abnormalities, structural defects such as spina bifida and anencephaly, and inherited metabolic disorders. Other common birth defects—congenital heart disorders, and cleft lip and palate, for example—and some types of mental retardation cannot be diagnosed, however. Amniocentesis, done late in the pregnancy, can also assess the maturity of the baby's lungs.

A woman thirty-five years or older can be virtually certain that her doctor will recommend amniocentesis. This now routine practice goes along with current medical thinking that women thirty-five or older are at increased risk of having a defective child. (Nancy Wainer Cohen and Lois J. Estner, in their book *Silent Knife* [South Hadley, Mass.: Bergin & Garvey, 1983], report that "British researchers suggest that only after 40 years of age is the indication for the procedure to detect an abnormality equal to or greater than the increased risk to the fetus.")

Clearly, then, the decision whether to have an amniocentesis is most difficult for women between the ages of thirty-five and forty, and is not helped by what some have called the procedure's major drawback—the timing. The medical protocol calls for amniocentesis to be done between the weeks 15 and 16 of pregnancy (with a few doctors now doing it as early as 12 to 14 weeks). It often takes up to an additional month to get the results. A small possibility exists, too, that the lab will ask for a repeat, involving even more waiting. If the test reveals a chromosome abnormality or other problem, the woman is faced with the decision of whether to go on with the pregnancy or face a late second-trimester abortion, which can be both emotionally and medically difficult. This leaves a very small window of decision-making opportunity.

Then there is the issue of accuracy and risks associated with the procedure itself. *Assuming an experienced doctor and technicians and a qualified lab to analyze the sample and calculate the results,* amniocentesis can be relatively accurate—the medical literature talks about nearly 100 percent accuracy. Just remember that only certain disorders can be detected by the procedure. So a "normal" finding does not guarantee a normal baby. And the procedure does carry some risks. There is a slight chance of a spontaneous abortion, or miscarriage—approximately 0.5 percent, according to recent findings—although other factors enter in here: past obstetric-gynecologic complications, mother's age and general health, and stage of pregnancy. Amniocentesis also carries a chance of introducing an infection, although the risk here is very low. A slim risk exists, too, for bleeding (less than 1 percent, says the American College of Obstetricians and Gynecologists) that ranges from the mild—spotting that lasts for only a day or so—to the more serious.

The latest research at Harvard Medical School suggests that women at high risk of having a baby with a neural tube defect—that is, women who have elevated levels of maternal serum alpha fetoprotein (see p. 103), according to the report in the *New England Journal of Medicine* (August 30, 1990)—can be screened just as well with ultrasound as with amniocentesis, which is more expensive and itself can cause miscarriage. In the article, the researchers emphasize that by sonography they are referring only to the more advanced "level 2" ultrasound exams done by specialists who can look for detailed fetal structures.

Ultrasound. At some point in the second trimester (usually between week 16 and week 18 or 20) your doctor may recommend an ultrasound to see that the fetus is developing normally. In this technique, sound waves are "bounced" off the baby's bones and other tissues to construct pictures showing shape and position. A technician passes what's called a transducer back and forth over the woman's abdomen, and a computer translates the resulting echoes into pictures on a television monitor. The image itself is called a sonogram. Taking usually not more than fifteen minutes, ultrasound is not invasive and does not involve X rays, and by and large the medical profession considers it safe—so certain of its benign nature that some doctors recommend all pregnant women have one done. More than one million scans are done annually on pregnant women, and a growing number of obstetrical offices are buying ultrasound equipment, especially because the doctors can be virtually certain that insurance companies will pick up the tab (that is, cover the services).

What has happened is that technology originally developed and recommended for high-risk situations has become almost routine in normal or borderline-suspicious pregnancies. Certainly, though, in certain pregnancies, especially high-risk ones, ultrasound has its uses:

- To detect pregnancies outside the uterus
- To detect multiple pregnancies (twins, triplets, and so on)
- To diagnose some fetal anomalies
- To guide in the performance of other diagnostic tests by showing the position of the fetus

111

Perhaps the fetus size does not correspond to the stage of the pregnancy, thus raising suspicions of intrauterine growth retardation, so the doctor orders an ultrasound. Or the doctor is being especially cautious because the woman's previous child was born with malformations or a disabling condition. Or maybe the doctor is afraid of malpractice suits and routinely orders extra tests—in short, practicing defensive medicine or "doing everything possible" in case something does go wrong.

Ask your doctor, "What will you be looking for in this ultrasound?" If the response you get is "I do it for all my patients—better safe than sorry," press your doctor for specifics. Or if the doctor says he wants to determine your "exact" due date (an increasingly popular pastime and a justification for an ultrasound), find out how precise the doctor wants to be and why. Also ask, "What about my unique condition makes this test worthwhile? What procedures or actions will be necessary or recommended if the ultrasound finds a problem?" Find out whether ultrasound is the most appropriate test and why, and discuss the relative perils and benefits. And, finally, ask, "What will happen if I don't have an ultrasound?" "What will happen if I wait?" "How will the results or information gained change anything?"

Before you can be certain of anything else, the sound waves you need here are verbal.

───── *Pregnancy and the Working Woman*

No doubt about it, the workplace can pose real dangers to the pregnant woman and the developing fetus. As we mentioned earlier, chemicals, gases, radiation, and infectious diseases are just a few of the hazards that affect not only your ability to become pregnant and to carry the pregnancy to term, but also the health of your baby. So scrutinizing your work environment with this in mind is smart. But what about the less dramatic dangers? Factors such as stress and deadline pressures; the amount of standing, lifting, and climbing involved in the job; or even the noise level in the office—what effects do they have on the healthy pregnancy and outcome?

For the safety of the mother and the fetus, how long should the pregnant woman continue working?

Until recently, the answer to the last question has been pretty much a guessing game. A doctor's dictums were based as much on myth and old wives' tales as anything else, but today, the climate of opinion (at least among the more enlightened souls) is that pregnancy is not an illness. And far from sheltering herself from the outside world, the pregnant woman, if she wishes, should continue to work and participate in many of the activities she engaged in before she was pregnant. But how far does she push that? Assuredly, every job is different, as are employer-provided disability plans, which also influence whether or not the woman works throughout her pregnancy.

In 1984, the American Medical Association's Council on Scientific Affairs issued guidelines on various types of work and how long a woman should continue to work in each job function, *assuming a normal, uncomplicated pregnancy.* After a review of scientific literature as of September 1988, the report was reissued with minor changes (see the chart on p. 114). Use these guidelines as the basis of discussions with your obstetrician and your employer—but remember (as even the report cautions): judgments on stopping or continuing work must be made on a case-by-case basis.

During the second trimester, you're typically seeing your doctor only every three to four weeks, and a large part of each visit is spent going through routine prenatal checks. So make the time count! Use your diary to jog your memory about concerns and questions you have.

What Are Some of the Common Problems?

No two pregnancies are alike, but certain discomforts are correspondent with the physical changes specific to the second trimester—increased blood volume, a swelling womb, weight gain, and the like. Some are

- edema, or water retention (primarily in feet, ankles, hands, fingers, and sometimes the face);
- nosebleeds and nasal congestion;

113

Guidelines for the Termination of Various Levels of Work During a Normal, Uncomplicated Pregnancy

Job Function	*Approximate Week of Gestation*
Secretarial and light clerical	40
Professional and managerial	40
Sitting with light tasks	
Prolonged (more than 4 hours)	40
Intermittent	40
Standing	
Prolonged (more than 4 hours)	24
Intermittent	
More than 30 minutes per hour	32
Less than 30 minutes per hour	40
Stooping and bending below knee level	
Repetitive	
More than 10 times per hour	20
Less than 2 times per hour	40
Climbing	
Vertical ladders and poles	
Repetitive Four times or more per 8-hour shift	28
Intermittent Less than 4 times per 8-hour shift	28
Stairs	
Repetitive Four times or more per 8-hour shift	28
Intermittent Less than 4 times per 8-hour shift	40
Lifting	
Repetitive	
More than 23 kg (about 50 lbs.)	20
Between 11 and 23 kg (25–50 lbs.)	24
Less than 11 kg (25 lbs.)	40
Intermittent	
More than 23 kg (about 50 lbs.)	30
Between 11 and 14 kg (25–30 lbs.)	40
Less than 11 kg (25 lbs.)	40

Source: Informational Report of the American Medical Association Council on Scientific Affairs, December 1988 (I-88), Book II.

Pregnancy Discrimination Act

Know Your Rights!

Not all the dangers to the pregnant woman in the workplace are tangible. Some lurk in the shadows, in the hearts and minds of employers and the benefits they allow (or disallow) pregnant workers. We're talking about discrimination, unfair treatment that includes prejudice against pregnant women in the workplace and outright inequality in pay and benefit schedules, promotions, and job security.

Some companies can be said to take advantage of the threat posed by toxins in the workplace to discriminate against pregnant women (or even all women of childbearing age). A Milwaukee company that makes automobile batteries is a good case in point. Citing the threat to reproductive health posed by the high concentrations of lead in the factory, the company barred women of childbearing age from some jobs—higher-paying jobs, said a suit filed by several women at the factory. In March 1991 the Supreme Court ruled in favor of the female employees. Critics of such so-called protective discrimination policies charge that women, faced with demotion or job loss, have opted to have themselves sterilized.

Fortunately, certain rights are guaranteed under the Pregnancy Discrimination Act, passed in 1978 as an amendment to Title VII of the 1964 Civil Rights Act, and they apply to every business that employs more than fifteen people:

● You cannot be refused a job, a promotion, or training because you are pregnant.
● You cannot be fired, demoted, or stripped of your seniority because you are pregnant.
● If you take a maternity leave, you are entitled to your same job, or one equivalent in pay and status to your old job, on the same basis as other employees who are disabled or take sick leave.
● If you are unable to work because of pregnancy, you are entitled to the same disability benefits as every other employee at your workplace.
● Employer health insurance plans must include coverage for pregnancy-related conditions.

(continued)

● hemorrhoids and varicose veins;
● leg cramps;
● gas, flatulence;
● breast enlargement and discharge; and
● increased salivation and perspiration.

Really more annoyances or discomforts than serious problems for most women, these concerns, nevertheless, should be

115

That's the good news; now for the bad. Unfortunately, maternity leave (beyond the interval of medical recovery), although a matter of major importance to working women who hope and plan to return to work, is *not* a universal right. Few states have specifically addressed the issue. In the vast majority of cases, it is the employer who determines the benefits. So if you desire extra time with your baby after you give birth—beyond the date your doctor says you are physically able to return to work—be prepared to negotiate.

But before you start the process, find out the experience of other co-workers and how they have handled their maternity leaves. If you have questions about your legal rights, the Equal Employment Opportunity Commission operates a hot line, in both English and Spanish. Call 1-800-USA-EEOC.

brought up in discussions with your doctor. (And remember, don't settle for "All pregnant women complain about something" or "That's all a part of being pregnant." This may be true, but an equal partnership relationship deserves a more supportive and thoughtful response.) Prevention is the best medicine, so ask your doctor what can be done to head these problems off at the pass. Just make sure your baby's safety is at the heart of any preventive approach. If prevention is impossible, find out what you can do to minimize discomfort. Wear support hose, for instance, to help with varicose veins. Or if water retention in your lower extremities is a problem, lie down with your feet raised a few times a day.

Braxton-Hicks Contractions

Now is a good time to talk about Braxton-Hicks contractions. Although they appear with greatest frequency and intensity late in the pregnancy, they can occur throughout the pregnancy, so you should be prepared in order to distinguish them from premature labor. They can confuse even the most experienced woman (and doctor, we might add).

Braxton-Hicks contractions are often called "false labor,"

although "practice labor" is probably more accurate because there is nothing false about the contractions—they're real. Braxton-Hicks contractions are mild, irregular uterine contractions, but they are of shorter duration than true labor contractions, usually lasting twenty to thirty seconds and generally stopping spontaneously after one or two hours (or perhaps even sooner if you change positions, walk around a bit, and so on). With Braxton-Hicks contractions, cervical dilation—widening of the cervix—never takes place.

In most cases, Braxton-Hicks contractions present no problem for the woman; they're just signs that the uterine muscles are tightening and loosening—some even call it practicing, as your body prepares for labor. Just make sure you (and your doctor) are straight on the general differences between these and true labor: what to look for in each. For instance, true labor usually occurs at regular intervals and with intensity that gradually increases, whereas Braxton-Hicks contractions are irregular and the intensity tends to remain the same. And the location of the discomfort may be different, too. Many describe the discomfort of true labor as predominantly in the back and abdomen, and in the lower abdomen for Braxton-Hicks contractions.

What Complications May Arise?

Cervical Incompetence. Cervical incompetence is the term the medical literature uses to describe an abnormality of the cervix that prevents it from performing its duty during pregnancy: keeping the fetus securely within the womb. The cervix dilates, or widens, instead of remaining tightly closed. Really one of a *weak* cervix, the condition, which may induce premature labor, may be caused by a trauma to the cervix or by a malformation, with the incidence of malformation higher in DES daughters. *Again, as we mentioned earlier with miscarriage, if your mother took DES when she was pregnant with you, then be sure to confer with your doctor on the possible repercussions for your own pregnancy.* The condition may be diagnosed ahead of time or during the pregnancy. Clearly, the earlier diagnosed, the better. Without treatment, most women with cervical incompetence do not carry to full term.

If undetected, the dilation of the cervix often results in a miscarriage, normally occurring during the second trimester. Ask your doctor what the early signs of dilation are—what you can look for: Is there any pain or discomfort? What preventive measures or treatments have been successful? Bed rest? When and for how long? What about cerclage—is this a viable option for you? Generally performed sometime after week 12 but not recommended in the third trimester, cerclage is the surgical closing of the cervix—literally a suture, or stitch, is what it takes. At around week 38, the stitch is removed, or right at the start of labor.

Gestational Hypertension. This is the hypertension, or high blood pressure, that may develop after week 20 of pregnancy. Fluctuations slightly above or even below some women's normal prepregnant levels are to be expected, but elevated blood pressure may be a sign of a more serious problem, impending preeclampsia, a toxic condition that can occur late in the pregnancy (see p. 120). Experts agree that the causes of gestational hypertension are little understood, although there is consensus that first pregnancies in women aged thirty-five or over carry a higher risk. In most cases, gestational hypertension resolves itself after the baby is born.

Meanwhile, there is reason enough to monitor your blood pressure closely throughout your pregnancy. If you are not already taking your own blood pressure at home, do it! Don't wait for your doctor to do it—that may be weeks away. Should your pressure be elevated, talk to your doctor about what you can do. In consultation with your doctor, determine how often you should take your blood pressure. Ask if you should reduce the salt intake in your diet. Contemporary thinking no longer considers it wise to eliminate salt during pregnancy, but in this case a minimal reduction may be called for. In severe cases, antihypertensive drugs have been used. Find out which, if any, your doctor recommends and get the lowdown on the drugs—usage, precautions, adverse reactions, dosages and administration, and so on—from the drug reference books we mentioned earlier (see p. 106). By all means discuss the relative

How High Is High?

Israeli research reported in the *New England Journal of Medicine* (August 10, 1989) defined pregnancy-induced hypertension as *systolic blood pressure* (the higher number) *in excess of 140 mm Hg,* and *diastolic blood pressure* (the lower number) *in excess of 90 mm Hg,* or both, when measured on at least two occasions within twenty-four hours of each other.

The Israeli study received a lot of attention for its findings that "low doses of aspirin [100 mg of acetylsalicylic acid, plus some fillers and binders] taken during the third trimester of pregnancy significantly reduce the incidence of pregnancy-induced hypertension preeclamptic toxemia in women at high risk for these disorders. . . ."

Another study, this one Italian and published in the same *New England Journal of Medicine* issue, "found that low-dose aspirin—60 mg per day from week 12 of gestation to delivery—given to women at risk for pregnancy-induced hypertension was associated with a longer duration of pregnancy and, more important, with an increase in the weight of the newborn." In the same breath, though, the researchers caution that *despite its potential benefit, the use of aspirin in pregnancy is not without risk.*

If you are experiencing gestational hypertension, obtain these reports (most local libraries either have or can get you a copy of the journal), show them to your physician, and discuss their application to you. Caution is the watchword, of course. The Israeli investigators pointed out that aspirin-sensitive women should steer clear of such therapy and "aspirin treatment [should] be stopped at least five days before the estimated date of delivery in order to minimize the risk of induced-bleeding disorders."

Don't start using aspirin without your doctor's advice. Because aspirin interferes with blood clotting, self-medication should be avoided.

risks and benefits. Don't enter lightly and uninformed into any drug regimen, even if it has the backing of your doctor, before you assess its safety during pregnancy.

Gestational Diabetes. This is a special short-term form of diabetes that can develop in a normally nondiabetic woman late in the second or early in the third trimester. Occurring in relatively few pregnancies—experts say some 1 to 3 percent—gestational diabetes can seriously jeopardize the health of your baby.

Excessive sugar in the urine, revealed through one of the routine urine tests you have at each office visit (or perhaps through home monitoring, too), can point to possible gestational diabetes, but absolute certainty is usually withheld until after results of blood sugar (glucose tolerance) testing. Experts cite the cost, duration, and inconvenience of the glucose tolerance test—factors that, they say, make it impractical to use on all pregnant women. Discuss this with your doctor. Should you have a glucose tolerance test? The opinion of many in the field is that you should have your urine checked twice in a row before getting a blood sugar (glucose tolerance) test.

If the blood sugar test is positive, what treatment options are open? Diet alone? (A technical review entitled "Diabetes and Pregnancy" in the journal *Medical Clinics of North America* [May 1989] reports that 85 percent of women with gestational diabetes can manage with diet alone, while only 10 to 15 percent require insulin during pregnancy.) And finally, if diet alone is the course you and your doctor agree on, ask about the necessity of follow-up weekly blood sugar tests until delivery.

Preeclampsia (or Toxemia of Pregnancy). First, a word about jargon: You're liable to read and hear a couple of different terms for this troublesome complication. Purists insist that preeclampsia refers to the milder form of toxemia, and eclampsia is the more severe, more advanced stage. Be sure you and your doctor are talking the same language.

After week 20 (some say week 24), some women develop high blood pressure, swelling of the face and hands, and protein in the urine. These symptoms may appear separately or together, and in random order; they may take several days to develop or appear quite suddenly over the course of twenty-four hours. In any event, *if you have any of these symptoms you should immediately consult your doctor.* Stock medical wisdom holds that *preeclampsia* is a prelude, in severe cases left untreated, to eclampsia: convulsions and even coma. Although preeclampsia occurs in relatively few pregnancies—

experts estimate somewhere around 5 percent of all pregnancies—it is a dangerous complication whose signs should not be ignored.

The cause of preeclampsia is not known, but there are risk factors. As your second trimester begins, talk to your doctor about any you may have—first pregnancy, age (under twenty or over forty years old), and history of high blood pressure, vascular disease, or kidney problems are just some mentioned in various sources. If you are at risk, should you step up the routine testing schedule—blood pressure, urine sampling, and the like? Is there anything you can do to prevent preeclampsia? (Many experts call good nutrition the best defense. Discuss specifics with your doctor, and if her knowledge of nutrition is inadequate, find someone who knows the ropes.) When does preeclampsia require hospitalization? How safe is drug therapy for preeclampsia and at what point is it resorted to? Are there any warning signs for eclampsia?

The Third Trimester: Weeks 27 through 40

The critical task in the last trimester is preparation for labor and delivery. And a very important part of this preparation is close attention to the growth and presentation of the baby.

What Is Presentation? Somewhere around week 26 and at every prenatal visit in the third trimester, your doctor will monitor the presentation, the "lie" or position, of the fetus. The fetus's presenting part is the part that is the first to emerge from the birth canal. Most babies adopt a head-down (called vertex or cephalic) presentation, the easiest way of delivery. Others have breech presentations—buttocks first, feet first, or whatever—although by the time of delivery, most who were in breech presentation at, say, week 32 or even later have turned themselves around.

Does a Breech Presentation Always Mean a Cesarean? You will want to discuss this issue with your doctor before your delivery date, because some doctors and hospitals still believe that an abnormal presentation necessitates a cesarean delivery. At every prenatal visit in the third trimester, ask the doctor what your baby's presentation is. Ask:

- Is the baby's head down?
- Back to my front?
- Crossways to me?
- A transverse lie?

If it is a breech presentation, and the baby has not turned naturally (by week 38, say the experts), ask about exercises you can do to help the baby turn. Also find out if the doctor is skilled in external cephalic version, a maneuver in which the practitioner tries to turn the baby from the outside. This requires specific skills and a delicacy of touch, and can be dangerous if performed by an inexperienced doctor.

Also discuss the baby's movement in the final two to four (or even six) weeks before delivery. Your doctor will probably talk about "lightening," or the fact that the baby has "dropped" or is "engaged." What does it all mean? When the doctor says the baby is "engaged," that means that the baby has dropped—its head has entered into your pelvis, a sign of a good position for birth. This is also known as "lightening" because of a certain lifting of pressure from your ribs and diaphragm that you may feel. When does this usually occur? Answers depend on a number of variables: for one, whether this is your first pregnancy or a subsequent one. In approximately half of first-time pregnancies, this occurs at around week 36—and in the others, some two weeks later. In subsequent pregnancies, it is not unusual for the head to engage as late as week 40 or right when labor begins. Talk to your doctor about this, and raise any questions you have in your childbirth preparation classes, too.

What Are the Signs of Labor? When Should You Call the Doctor, Perhaps Even Proceed to Your Chosen Birth Setting? "Don't worry, you'll know" is not the response you're looking for. After all your planning, discussing, and negotiating, you may not want to go to the hospital (if that's the birth setting you've chosen) any earlier than you need to—many experts believe that rather typical predicament tends to place a woman at greater risk of a cesarean delivery. But neither do you want to dillydally when there's work to be done.

Incorporate into your discussions about the baby's movement and presentation specific questions about labor. Most assuredly, labor is a distinctly unique experience, varying from woman to woman and even from a woman's first childbirth to her subsequent ones. Nevertheless, you can talk about topics such as the rupture of the membranes (or "breaking of the bag of waters"). Does that mean labor is imminent? (Experts do agree that any leakage or gush of fluid, whether on schedule or not, is reason to call the doctor.) What are the stages in which labor usually occurs? (The first begins with contractions and ends when the cervix is fully dilated, or widened. The second starts when the cervix is dilated to its fullest—about ten centimeters, or four inches—and ends with the delivery of the baby. The third stage starts with the baby's delivery and ends when the placenta is expelled.) Is there a typical duration of each? Ask about contractions—magnitude, rhythm, frequency, and duration.

Also talk about the dilation of the cervix—what's expected and when. Don't be surprised when more jargon creeps in. For instance, your doctor will mention effacement. That refers to the thinning or flattening of the cervix as it is drawn up by contractions until it becomes continuous with the lower part of the uterus. Transition, which you've probably heard other women talk about in no uncertain terms, is the end of the first stage of labor, when the cervix is fully dilated. It is often described as the most difficult part of labor. Remember, though, that most childbirth preparation programs stress the part you play at each stage and also which breathing and relaxation techniques to employ.

And finally, what complications *during* labor should you be aware of? Preparation, even for these, is the best medicine, because you're less likely to panic if you are familiar with the potential problems such as prolonged or difficult labor. Of course, by this time in your pregnancy, you should have questioned your birth practitioner on all the hard issues: the question of induction and stimulation of labor; the use of painkillers and anesthesia; the indications for cesarean delivery; the questionable necessity of episiotomy versus preventive mea-

123

sures; and the like. So you and your doctor should be squared away on your preferences.

── *What Complications May Arise?*

Antepartum hemorrhage is the medical term for heavy vaginal bleeding in the third trimester. Two late-pregnancy complications can cause severe bleeding: *abruptio placentae* or *placenta previa.*

Abruptio Placentae (or Placental Separation). In this condition, anywhere from the sixth month to the end of pregnancy—either prematurely, or close to or at term—suddenly the placenta partially separates or completely detaches from the uterine wall. The primary warning signs, bleeding and cramping, can be either mild or severe, depending on the degree of separation. In the case of complete detachment—or severe cases when half or more of the placenta separates—there may be considerable blood loss and abdominal pain, but not necessarily in every case. The blood may remain hidden in the uterine cavity.

Any sign of bleeding in the third trimester is a signal to call your doctor immediately or go to the emergency room. Ask your doctor in your routine visits during the last trimester: Can strenuous activity, sexual intercourse, or exercise cause it? What about a fall? If you should experience any of the symptoms, what tests or procedures does your doctor recommend? Does placental separation bring on premature labor? When is bleeding severe enough to merit a transfusion? When is hospitalization necessary? Or simply bed rest? When is an emergency cesarean section necessary?

Placenta Previa. This is a placenta that is abnormally low in the womb and that either partially or completely covers the opening of the cervix. It results when the fertilized egg, rather than implanting itself in the proper place—the upper portion of the womb—drops and implants itself in the lower half. Sometimes the placenta starts off too low in the womb, but as the pregnancy develops, it moves up the wall of the uterus to a more appropriate placement. A relatively rare occurrence, *placenta previa* occurs in approximately 1 in 200 to 1 in 250 pregnancies, usually the first pregnancy. Depending on its severity, the condition can lead to premature birth or stillbirth, and in certain cases cesarean delivery is mandated. Painless vaginal bleeding is the primary symptom.

Discuss this complication with your doctor, and ask questions until you're sure you know what it is, what to look for, and what to do and when. Is there always bleeding? How early can you diagnose this condition? With what tests? Is normal labor ever possible? When is hospitalization necessary? Or simply bed rest? When is an emergency cesarean section necessary?

There can be other complications of late pregnancy:

- *Preterm, or premature, labor* begins before the due date—indeed, sometimes long before it. The medical literature usually terms any birth before week 20 a miscarriage, and between weeks 20 and 37 prematurity. As you might imagine, the onset of contractions is a typical sign, but ask your doctor about any other warning signs, such as backache and pelvic pressure, spotting, or bleeding. And, again, remember to talk to her about the difference between true premature labor and Braxton-Hicks contractions. Discuss the risk factors for premature labor—such as DES exposure in utero, a history of preterm delivery, and maternal age—and whether you yourself are at risk. Are there activities you should refrain from (or any you should be doing) in the hope of preventing preterm labor? What about hospitalization and/or bed rest—when are they recommended?

- *Premature rupture of membranes* is the leakage of amniotic fluid before labor has begun. Premature breaking of the waters may be followed by premature labor. Even if not, premature rupture can be a problem for the fetus who is no longer protected by the amniotic fluid. It is difficult to generalize about treatment because it depends on the woman's situation—how many pregnancies she's had, how close to full term the pregnancy is, and other factors. For instance, if the membranes rupture too early, before week 35, your doctor may try to delay labor in order to give the fetus more time to develop and ma-

125

ture. In this case, if infection (a potential complication with premature rupture) can be prevented, you may be kept in bed and monitored carefully until labor occurs spontaneously. Or, if there are signs of infection, your doctor may induce labor or perform a cesarean section.

So be sure your doctor details what to look for, what to do, and the typical medical plan of action to prevent further complications.

● *Postmaturity* is the prolongation of pregnancy beyond when the baby is fully mature and able to survive on its own—some experts specify beyond week 42. The motivation for much additional testing and often a source of great stress for the woman, postmaturity is an issue you must discuss with your doctor. How long is "too long" overdue? What tests does she recommend, why, and when? When is artificial induction of labor recommended versus a wait-and-see attitude?

What If You Go Beyond Your Due Date? What Tests Will Your Doctor Recommend?

Nonstress Test. This is a test using external fetal monitoring that a doctor often recommends when she is uncertain as to fetal movement and other high-risk problems such as a prolonged pregnancy. Using ultrasound, the test permits the fetal heart rate and fetal movement to be monitored and correlated. The doctor is looking for assurance that the baby, for instance, is receiving enough oxygen or that the nervous system is functioning well, but many sources report that not every doctor has the same standards for a normal response. And, of course, a nonreactive baby doesn't necessarily mean that the baby is in danger. Discuss all this with your doctor.

Stress Test. Sometimes called the oxytocin challenge test (OCT), this test stimulates the uterus with Pitocin (a synthetic form of oxytocin, a natural hormone secreted during childbirth) and determines the effect of contractions on fetal heart rate. The stress test (usually recommended after the nonstress test indicates potential problems) seeks to determine the same

Intrauterine Death

Although definitions vary, most physicians define *intrauterine death* as the term for death of a fetus in the uterus after week 20. (Spontaneous abortion, or miscarriage, is usually defined as the loss of a pregnancy before week 20.) Regular fetal movement is one of the easiest ways to determine fetal well-being, along with fetal heartbeat, of course. Although fetal movement begins somewhere around week 12, it isn't until around weeks 18 to 20 that the mother is actually aware of the movements. As soon as you discover you're pregnant, ask your doctor what sensations to expect throughout the course of your pregnancy. Doctors differ on exactly what you should be feeling, when, and how often—but the general consensus seems to be that any long period (two or more days) between fetal movements should be reported to your practitioner. Although this may turn out to be normal, the fact that you may not have certain sensations should lead you to further discussions and perhaps testing. In the absence of a fetal heartbeat, for example, a fetal ultrasound may be ordered to determine whether the fetus is alive.

The consensus is that most fetuses deliver spontaneously soon after demise. Studies have indicated that the range is somewhere between the end of the second to the end of the third week following the death. But this is not always the case. There are times when a fetus has died but has not been expelled for four weeks or more, thus posing medical, not to mention psychological, problems for the mother. The key question for you and your doctor to discuss is whether to await the onset of spontaneous labor or have labor induced.

thing as the nonstress—in this case, whether the baby's heart rate remains stable even during contractions, whether the baby can withstand the "stress" of labor. Critics of this test cite high false-positive rates and a tendency to misinterpret results, and they call it an unnatural intervention, one that can lead to artificial induction of labor for a baby not yet ready to be born.

For some authorities, the safest and easiest (and least costly, we might add) way to assess how the baby will manage during labor is by stimulation of the mother's nipples. This causes her to release oxytocin, which in turn stimulates uterine contractions. The mother's contractions and the baby's heart rate are then measured.

—— How Will You Know When Labor Has Begun?

As we discuss in more depth in Chapter 6, preparation for childbirth is probably the most important issue during pregnancy. If you and your partner prepare, you will go into labor and delivery informed, and knowing what to expect and when. Every woman's labor is different—no two are exactly alike—but there are some tried-and-true signs of impending labor. No doubt your childbirth preparation instructor will tell you about them, as will your birth practitioner. But here's a quick rundown:

- *Engagement.* This is when the fetus is beginning to settle into the birth canal. Many women attest to feeling less pressure on their lungs and say they can "breathe easier" than they have in the earlier stages of pregnancy.

- *Extraordinary Burst of Energy.* Not every woman experiences this, of course, but it forms the core of the so-called old wives' tale that the urge to mop the kitchen floor or undertake some other project is a sign.

- *Bloody Show.* Late in the pregnancy, your cervix begins to shorten and thin out (efface). Right before labor or just as it begins, many women notice a slightly blood-tinged mucous discharge. This indicates that the small plug that seals the cervix has come out.

- *Rupture of the Membranes (Breaking of Waters).* Not every woman experiences this—the rupture of the amniotic sac that contains the amniotic fluid—but if you do, don't necessarily expect a rush of water. For some, the rupture involves a mere trickle of fluid, usually clear (or sometimes milky) and odorless. Most birth practitioners believe that the woman should notify her chosen practitioner when this occurs, because labor generally starts within twelve or so hours.

- *Contractions.* As mentioned before, Braxton-Hicks contractions often occur throughout the pregnancy, increasing in frequency and intensity in the third trimester. So, to many experts' way of thinking, contractions are not necessarily a reliable sign of labor because they can be misleading. That's why we have stressed the importance of discussing with your doctor the difference between true labor and Braxton-Hicks contractions. Some women (and practitioners) want to wait to go to the hospital or the birthing center until the contractions become more frequent and strong. This is certainly a key topic for you and your doctor to cover. What you *don't* want is an unplanned home birth!

    Remember too, the three distinct stages of labor:

- Stage 1, which starts with the beginning of contractions and ends with full dilation of the cervix (10 cm, or 4 inches)
- Stage 2, which begins with the full dilation and ends with the birth of the baby
- Stage 3, which begins with the birth of the baby and ends with the expulsion, or delivery, of the placenta.

    Just as with pregnancy, labor is different for every woman, but you can certainly be prepared and informed, ready to make decisions as the need arises.

CHAPTER SIX

The Birth

Preparation for Childbirth

Although there is no way to know what childbirth is *really* like except by going through it, of course, knowledge is power—and the best defense against fear and pain, say childbirth educators. The idea here is to familiarize yourself with the events associated with labor, in its various stages, and delivery; learn how to help yourself during these stages, through breathing and relaxation techniques; and have your partner learn how to help, too. But as with so many other things associated with your pregnancy, there are varied methods and approaches, so give yourself time to check around for the program that best meets your needs.

A Brief Overview of the "Revolution in the Delivery Room"

Pioneering the earliest theories of "natural childbirth," as it came to be called, was a British physician named Grantly Dick-Read whose work led him to conclude that fear is the major source of pain in childbirth. Women, he said, are culturally conditioned to fear childbirth; that fear in turn creates a tension, which then produces pain, thus causing even more tension and pain. Education and knowledge, in combination with physical awareness, breathing control, and relaxation techniques, will eliminate fear and enable most women to deliver comfortably without anesthesia. Dick-Read's classic work *Childbirth Without Fear*, published in 1944, set forth his ideas on this fear-tension-pain cycle, the principles and practices behind which remained popular in the United States through the 1950s.

The term *natural childbirth*, which Dick-Read used in the title of another book, suffered some discredit when it became synonymous with nonmedication and "brave suffering," even martyrdom. Certainly apt if you consider a drugged stupor to be an unnatural state in which to give birth, the term *natural childbirth* fell from favor partly because Dick-Read and other proponents made room in their philosophy for the benefits of modern birth technology and also because the medical profession did its best to associate the idea of "natural" with "primitive" and "dangerous." Nowadays, the early theories are more likely to go under the term *prepared childbirth*. (Note: *family-centered childbirth*, another popular term, may be close to the same thing—the idea that the woman through education and awareness of breathing and relaxation techniques can actively participate in labor and delivery—or it may be merely a marketing term. Be sure to find out whether it truly is a method that allows you options and control or a method to lure you into the standard hospital childbirth routine.)

At the same time, but independent of Dick-Read's work, a French obstetrician named Fernand Lamaze was studying Pavlov's conditioned response theory and a Russian method to reduce pain in childbirth. Back in Paris in the early 1950s, he introduced his method "childbirth without pain"—*accouchement sans douleur*—and wrote in his 1956 book *Painless Childbirth* that a woman can *learn* how to give birth without pain. Also called psychoprophylaxis because of the psychological prevention of pain it involves, the Lamaze method employs *controlled* breathing and concentration on specific distracting stimuli (for example, staring at a focal point, or "spot") to block sensations of pain. It also encourages the idea of labor support or coaching.

While the method advocates unmedicated hospital childbirth, the use of drugs is not forbidden in the practice of Lamaze in this country, a fact that some say goes far in explaining the method's widespread acceptance among doctors and hospitals.

Thanks in part to Marjorie Karmel, the Lamaze method was introduced in America, grew more popular, and eventually replaced the Dick-Read method, whose "rhapsodic and mystical view of childbirth," as Karmel described it, became increasingly out of place with changing attitudes and times. Karmel's book *Thank You, Dr. Lamaze*, first published in 1959, describes her own experiences of giving birth in France and of her later efforts to find a doctor in New York who would help her give birth using the Lamaze method. A magazine article Karmel wrote on the same subject attracted the attention of European-trained physical therapist Elisabeth Bing, who, along with medical professionals in 1960, founded the American Society for Psychoprophylaxis in Obstetrics (ASPO) to promote acceptance of the Lamaze method. (Bing also is the author of *Six Practical Lessons for an Easier Childbirth*, heralded as a guide and supplement to childbirth preparation classes but also valuable as a complete home course in neuromuscular-control exercises, or concentration and relaxation exercises.)

From its early origins, ASPO branched out, reorganized to give three coalitions equal board representation and voting power—physicians, other professionals (mostly childbirth educators), and parents—and now certifies instructors (most of whom come from backgrounds in nursing or physical therapy) to teach Lamaze preparation classes for parents.

Even with critics both inside and outside medical circles, the Lamaze method has undergone a number of modifications to keep it up to date and today remains the most well known and widely used method of prepared childbirth.

Another name in prepared childbirth is Robert A. Bradley, who used Dick-Read's principles but broadened the approach to include the concept of "husband-coached" childbirth. In fact, that is the title of his influential book, first published in 1965, the idea behind which is that the baby's father—his presence, support, and coaching—are unequivocally necessary throughout labor and delivery. "Bradley supplied 'the missing piece' to family-centered maternity care," states Constance A. Bean in the revised edition of her own classic book *Methods of Child-birth* (New York: Morrow, 1990).

The Bradley method emphasizes the six conditions paralleled in the animal world that the delivering woman requires to give birth naturally in the hospital: darkness and solitude; quiet; physical comfort; physical relaxation; controlled breathing; and closed eyes and the appearance of sleep. A radical departure from the Lamaze method is Bradley's avowed goal of a totally unmedicated delivery. Claiming to be the only preparation for a truly and entirely natural childbirth, the Bradley method is taught by the American Academy of Husband-Coached Childbirth.

The final installment in childbirth preparation methods we will talk about was introduced by Sheila Kitzinger, an English anthropologist. Set forth in her 1962 book *The Experience of Childbirth*, her major contribution to the revolution (or evolution, whichever you prefer) in the delivery room was to describe childbirth as and parallel it with a personal, sexual event. She also incorporates relaxation, breathing, and the necessity of comfortable positions for labor. While her "psychosexual" approach, as it has been called, is not actually a method because there is no Kitzinger organization or instructors, many of her ideas have been incorporated into other prepared childbirth teachings: namely, the psychology of pregnancy, mental imagery to enhance relaxation, and massage.

In the 1970s, the French obstetrician Frederick Leboyer, in his film *Gentle Birth* and book *Birth Without Violence*, both classics, raised our awareness and consciousness about the treatment of newborn babies. Rather than the brisk efficiency exemplified by forceps delivery and the rough treatment necessary to revive a drugged baby, Leboyer advocated immersing the newborn in warm water, thereby enabling the baby to move around freely in an environment similar to its comfortable uterine "home." Nowadays, in birth settings that follow Leboyer's teachings, gentle massage and skin-to-skin contact with the mother have replaced immersion, calm and quiet have replaced clanking metal noises that disturb the newborn, and procedures such as suctioning the infant are avoided.

Hardly a conclusive list, but representative of the major

movements that shaped thinking, the various childbirth preparation methods discussed above are taught all over the country—and they comprise the approaches that many people continue to lump under the term *natural childbirth* or *prepared childbirth*. All developed, in one way or another, out of the belief that unnecessary medical interventions and the laboring woman's fear and ignorance can lead to complications and that awake, participatory childbirth places the reins of control back where they belong—in the woman's hands.

Choose your childbirth educator as carefully as you would choose a doctor, and make sure that your attitudes and preferences are compatible with the teacher's, because only then will childbirth preparation truly prepare you to achieve your goals. And really good, thorough childbirth education is healthy for both you and your baby. Along with providing diet and exercise tips, it should prepare you to avoid merely routine obstetric interventions that have no medical necessity, to understand the physiological changes that occur during the course of pregnancy, and to understand and prepare for all aspects of labor and delivery. Be aware that not every doctor or hospital is joyous at the prospect of an informed, prepared couple—this is usually because either the doctor or the hospital (or both) consciously or unconsciously desire to thwart the couple's plans, regain control, and steer the childbirth into the high-tech routine many medicos have come to know and love. Don't let that happen—be prepared!

How to Choose a Childbirth Preparation Program

- *Decide what type of childbirth experience you want and find the method and course that will prepare you for it.* For instance, if you are adamantly against pain-relief medications, and do not consider them "tools to aid labor," as they have been called, but absolutely a last resort, then don't waste any time before asking what the program's attitudes are toward this issue. Valmai Howe Elkins, herself a childbirth educator for many years, says that many courses teach "what to do until you have your epidural" (*The Rights of the Pregnant Parent*), so avoid these if you are aiming specifically for unmedicated childbirth. And go beyond merely the name of the method. As popular and widespread as the Lamaze method is, many classes may be marketed under that name—maybe with a lowercase *L*—when they actually combine approaches or just use the name for recognition appeal. If you specifically want an American Society for Psychoprophylaxis in Obstetrics/Lamaze–sponsored course or a Bradley method instructor, for example, then contact the appropriate organization for referrals, or you can ask to see the instructor's credentials (background, training, and experience).

- *Decide what you want from the classes.* Do you want a truly couple-oriented program, your partner present at every class? Your partner present for only a few sessions? A woman-centered approach—you alone? When do you want to begin childbirth education classes? Do you want the standard timing— that is, later in the pregnancy—or do you want to start with early pregnancy classes? Usually offered within the first few months and perhaps as late as the sixth month, early pregnancy classes differ from childbirth preparation because they do not get into labor and delivery but instead focus on the early and ongoing physical and emotional changes. Ask if there is a refresher course, should you feel the need to bone up on your techniques between the last regular class and your due date.

  Do you want hospital-sponsored classes or private classes? (You should realize, though, that hospital classes may be "contracted out," either to a private instructor or to a private childbirth education association. Be sure to ask about this.) Your doctor will probably recommend the course given by the hospital (or the doctor even may have a childbirth educator on staff right there in the office), and many women and couples automatically go along with this because they do not know that there are independent childbirth educators who are not affiliated with any doctor or hospital. Or they do not know that there are national organizations that certify childbirth educators and will make referrals. True, there may be advantages to the hospital-sponsored course—maybe the instructor is an obstetric nurse and can "tell it like it is" (whether she is trained in teaching methods and childbirth education is another matter and whether she will be objective is extremely doubtful), and you are right where you will be on delivery day so you can familiarize yourself with the hospital and surroundings.

Rather than feeling reassured by the hospital presence, however, a lot of people are uncomfortable because they feel that the instruction—either blatantly or covertly—ignores options outside the hospital routine and protocol. In general, private classes tend to be smaller, more informal, and more objective about community medical services and practices. And you don't (or shouldn't) have to attend hospital-sponsored classes in order to have a tour of the maternity unit.

- *Call around.* If the hospital- or doctor-sponsored course is not for you, you must explore the other options available. But to save time and unnecessary running around, do the initial questioning and interviewing by telephone. Consult your Yellow Pages ("childbirth education" and "parent education" are good places to start), call the local La Leche League chapter and women's centers, check your newspaper for community courses such as the YWCA often offers, contact national organizations that provide childbirth education materials, and talk to public health nurses and midwives in your community. Ask around, too— the other women or couples in the doctor's waiting room, your friends, and so on.

These are the leading national organizations with childbirth educator certification programs, and most also give referrals:

American Academy of Husband-Coached Childbirth
    P.O. Box 5224
    Sherman Oaks, California 91413
    Telephone: 1-800-42-BIRTH (in California); 1-818-788-6662

American Society for Psychoprophylaxis in Obstetrics/Lamaze
    1101 Connecticut Avenue, N.W., Suite 300
    Washington, D.C. 20036
    Telephone: 1-202-857-1128

Cesarean Prevention Movement, Inc.
    University Station
    P.O. Box 152
    Syracuse, New York 13210
    Telephone: 1-315-424-1942

International Childbirth Education Association
P.O. Box 20048
Minneapolis, Minnesota, 55420
Telephone: 1-612-854-8660

Read Natural Childbirth Foundation, Inc.
P.O. Box 150956
San Rafael, California 94915
Telephone: 1-415-456-8462

To find a childbirth preparation teacher/program that emphasizes alternative methods of childbirth, your best bet is to contact:

National Association of Parents and Professionals for Safe
Alternatives in Childbirth
Route 1, Box 646
Marble Hill, Missouri 63764
Telephone: 1-314-238-2010

- *Have the program send a syllabus or its packet of materials used in the classes.* Here you are checking to see if the topics covered match your desires and expectations. How consumer-oriented is the material? Are diet and nutrition included? Information on breast-feeding, newborn care, and other postpartum issues? Emphasis on cesarean prevention? A scheduled tour of a hospital? Breathing and relaxation techniques and other exercises? What is the format? Lecture or group and individual participation? Ideally, the format should include both—some time spent in discussion followed by, say, an hour spent practicing techniques and exercises. Also within the packet of materials should be the instructor's credentials, maybe even recommendations from others who have taken the course. If not, ask.

- *Arrange to sit in on a session.* Does the reality match the verbal description or promotional pamphlet? Is it truly a small, interactive group or a too-large-to-be-effective size?

- *Find out the cost and arrangements for payment.* Generally, all courses, even hospital-sponsored programs, involve a fee, even though you would think that hospitals would have childbirth education as part of their primary mission. To see if you will get your money's (and time's) worth, break down the cost per lesson or per hour. Are audiovisual aids (slides, films, and videotapes) used? Printed handouts such as a class manual? Is there a lending library of books for your use?

- *Shop around for a suitable childbirth education program as early as possible in your pregnancy.* And be sure to inform your doctor of your choice, the topics, and so on. Remember, even though you may have found *the* approach for you, you *still* need a supportive doctor.

You cannot have the childbirth experience you desire if you do not know how the system works at the setting you and your doctor have chosen, how to negotiate with your doctor before your delivery day, and what strategies to employ *once there* to counteract any momentum running contrary to the choices you and your doctor agreed on in advance.

How to Have the Childbirth You Want

Last-Minute Arrangements

There are always last-minute arrangements to be made before any endeavor. The end of your pregnancy is no different because it truly is the start of another journey that entails even more things to think about and more arrangements you need to make before you go. Just as all the preliminary steps were empowering—choosing the right practitioner, birth setting, and childbirth preparation program; and reading, questioning, and investigating—so, too, are these arrangements. They are crucial to your well-being and the amount of control you have over your childbirth experience.

- As the date approaches, *continue to work out with your doctor specific details* of how you expect the birth to be handled. And don't take anything for granted. Of course, negotiating in advance is preferential—baby's father or other companion present throughout labor, delivery, and recovery; no shaving of pubic area; no sedatives, tranquilizers, analgesics, or anesthetics unless medically necessary and only with your approval; alternative treatment in the event of slow or long labor; spontaneous rupture of waters; varied birth positions (other than lithotomy) tried to see what works best; and so on. And these should long ago have been discussed, negotiated, agreed on, and listed in your birth plan. Even if you already discussed with your doctor what you want as well as routine treatment you don't want, do it again as you get closer to your due date.

When we earlier advised that you get all this in writing, we meant it. Have the list attached to your medical record at the doctor's office, make sure your doctor attaches it to your preadmission hospital forms, and bring a copy of the list with you to the hospital when you check in. Keep one at your side, and wave it in the face of every new person you encounter (remember, shift changes mean personnel changes). Here again—don't take anything for granted. Sure, your doctor may agree with your birth preferences, but your doctor probably is not going to be available to confirm all your requests until right before delivery.

- *Don't consent in advance to anything.* You have the right to informed consent—simply put, this is the idea that you have the right to available information about your condition and about the benefits and risks of procedures the doctors want to perform on you. Then you can make an informed decision about what is done to your body and your life before you give the go-ahead or refusal. Usually along with all the preadmission papers shoved in front of you to sign is a standard, or "blanket," consent form. (If not at the doctor's office, then the forms are there at the hospital or birthing center waiting for you or the baby's father to sign. But caution your partner to minimize the time spent jumping through these bureaucratic hoops so that you are not left alone.) This is not exactly an informed-consent situation, because although you are doing a whole load of consenting, they are not doing any informing. By signing a blanket consent form, you are in essence saying "Do with me as you will. I am giving up all rights to make decisions, to say no, or to sue you if you do me harm." In one short form, your rights are negated.

  Instead, sign the form—but only after you have added to or modified it to your liking. This is the time to be sensitive to and assertive (again!) about your choices, those preferences you, your doctor, and probably your partner agreed on way back at the dawn of the pregnancy or after numerous discussions. Note the items to which you take specific and strong objection. If the doctor's receptionist or assistant says you can't add statements to the form, then speak to the doctor. If the admissions person balks, your partner/advocate should ask to see the admissions director or another administrator—who will probably let you do whatever you want with the form because she will know that such blanket rights–robbers are more than likely indefensible in a court of law. They just use these forms, it seems, to keep the uninformed and easily intimidated in line. You, instead, should use it as an "escape hatch," in the words of a noted childbirth educator.

- *Just say no.* In reality, no matter how many forms you sign, no matter what you agree to, you have the right to refuse treatment. And if necessary—you're probably going to be busy and very focused during labor and delivery when apparatus-toting, intervention-minded hospital personnel come around— let your partner/coach do the nay-saying. And every time you or your coach says no, that forces the birth attendants to explain things to you so that you can make informed decisions.

- *Don't take no for an answer.* You're the captain of the team, the CEO, the head honcho, the principal player. Whatever you want to call it, you're in charge. It's your pregnancy, your childbirth, and, finally, your baby.

Discussing Controversial Issues with Your Doctor Ahead of Time

Major areas of controversy exist in obstetrics, both *within* the profession as well as between consumers and medical traditionalists. The fact that the United States has about a 25 percent cesarean-section rate is one—England considers its 11 percent rate a crisis—and the use of sonograms, medications during pregnancy, forceps, and episiotomy are just a few of the other disputable issues a woman must deal with before, during, and even after childbirth. The surest way to avoid routine (rather than mandatory) medicine is to know what the medical interventions are and their risks and benefits. Take the point of view that an intervention *will be used* if you do not negotiate with your doctor (the obstetrician being the main culprit here) to prevent its use! Not uncommonly, the doctor's attitude is something like "You may think you know what you *want*, but I know what you *need*" or, worse yet, the doctor may imply that by questioning the necessity of routine practices—the electronic fetal monitor, for one—you are not quite as concerned about the baby as you should be.

A particularly revealing and perhaps even typical account of such an attitude—unbeknownst to the doctor/writer, we might add—is an article in a popular medical magazine, *Medical Economics* (September 18, 1989). The article, "Winning Over a Patient Who Balks at Your Treatment," tells the doctors/readers that the dogmatic "I'm the doctor, do what I say" approach is bad for business and suggests other methods of accomplishing the same goal—patient compliance and passivity. But the initial paragraphs really set the tone:

> Paralleling the scientific advances in medicine these days has been the rise of a new breed of informed and often demanding health care consumers—patients who take exception to our treatment regimens and make it difficult to provide what we believe is the best care.
>
> As an [ob-gyn] specialist, I've become especially familiar with this problem. Massive media coverage is often critical of the techniques we accept as necessary for proper [obstetric] care. As a result, the gravid [pregnant] patient and her partner tend to specify how they want their baby brought into the world.

Most assuredly, this is not the medical mind-set of every doctor or even of yours. But you should know that there are plenty of others just like this. Don't bow to attitudes or implications of this sort. Use a birth plan for discussion and negotiation, and do it as soon as possible—that way, you have ample time to shop around for another birth practitioner if *the doctor* balks at *your* ideas and choices.

Unfortunately, many women are subjected to birth procedures or techniques that are more a matter of routine hospital policy than sound medical practice. Many of these obstetric practices result from the system of medical training that emphasizes intervention in or aggressive treatment of pregnancy and childbirth. Know and recognize the common interventions in childbirth, and discuss them way ahead of time with your physician, because the *labor and delivery rooms are not the optimum settings in which to lobby most effectively for the childbirth experience you desire.*

Standard Prepping

Shave, enema, and intravenous feeding (IV) comprise what's called "standard prepping" or standard obstetric admitting procedures. Some hospitals do these routinely, some do not, and others offer the procedures as options. Before you report to the hospital, if that's the setting you've chosen, you should already have discussed what procedures are in common use there, but even if you have made prior arrangements *not* to have these done, don't assume that every hospital employee who comes in is going to know or obey your wishes. Have the doctor put your wishes in his orders, which should be at the hospital when you arrive, but even with your doctor backing your choices, he is probably not going to be in the hospital, at your side, throughout the entire labor and delivery. So make the attending staff refer to the orders if questions arise. You and your partner also should practice your nay-saying because hospital routines otherwise have a way of snowballing—and rolling over you.

Sometimes just the shave of the pubic area is called a "prep," the justification for which is that shaving reduces infection. *Au contraire*, says the research; in actuality, not only is a shave a minor, unnecessary discomfort to the woman in labor, but it also may increase the woman's chances of infection—presumably from tiny razor nicks, which allow passage of bacteria or viruses.

Enemas, so goes the medical myth, are needed to clean out the woman's bowel so that there's no worry about fecal contamination as she's giving birth. The fallacy here is that nature typically takes care of that, and bowels often empty of their own just prior to labor. Another viewpoint is to have the woman give herself an enema—be sure to discuss the specifics with your doctor—in the privacy and comfort of her home before she goes to the hospital. Far from benign, an enema is an uncomfortable experience, just disruptive and irritating enough to make the most relaxed woman become tense. And for many women already in active labor, the enema can make contractions stronger and more uncomfortable, thus triggering demands for drugs.

A more recent addition to the standard procedures, an IV—in which an intravenous pathway is inserted into the woman's arm—is rationalized this way: IV feeding allows fluids to be given to prevent dehydration and depletion in the fasting woman (the withholding of food and water being another hospital routine); it is useful "just in case" emergency anesthesia or painkilling or labor-augmenting drugs must be administered; and it is necessary if a woman goes into shock and her veins collapse, thus making it difficult to start an IV. But the consensus of opinion is that the normal labor and delivery probably do not require the intervention, which itself may cause infection at the site of insertion—not to mention the fact that the IV hookup is uncomfortable and impedes movement. Other experts maintain that IV feeding may not even supply adequate and proper nutritional support to the woman in labor.

Frankly, the entire idea of fasting has come under criticism, especially since IV feeding is no substitute for appropriate foods and fluids, assuming the woman is not vomiting and can eat and drink. After all, labor is work, and work requires energy. In the medical scheme, the rationale behind fasting is that it is necessary should general anesthesia be required. In other words, here's yet another obstetric practice that pushes the *low-risk* pregnant woman one step closer to becoming *high risk* by removing an obstacle to intervention. Discuss with your doctor the possibility of having light food and clear liquids during labor.

A final problem, as more than one critic of the procedure has pointed out, is that an IV hookup makes it more difficult for the woman (and her partner) to monitor what goes into her body through the needle. Are drugs being given—and are they wanted or needed, or are they just a part of the doctor's "standing orders"?

Confinement to bed has always been standard procedure for the heavily sedated laboring woman. But what about the woman who is fully awake? Why is she not encouraged to remain ambulatory in labor? Critics of the horizontal (or supine or lithotomy, as the medicos call it) birthing position—giving birth while lying flat on a table—say that it lengthens labor (thus paving the way for painkilling or labor-augmenting drugs); interferes with blood circulation; may cause a drop in blood pressure and thus lowers oxygen supply to the baby; and heightens the atmosphere of debility surrounding hospital childbirth. They declare that, by making the woman work against gravity, the supine position is unnatural—indeed, it is hard to find a worse position for labor and delivery. Research has found that an upright position actually reduces the length of labor by more than an hour (*Ob. Gyn. News*, July 15–31, 1985) and reduces maternal trauma, such as vaginal tears, during delivery.

Why, then, do so many doctors and hospitals persist in putting the healthy woman, with a normal pregnancy, to bed and then require that she deliver flat on her back with her legs up in the air? We have already seen how the supine position clears the way for other interventions: drugs, episiotomy, forceps, to name a few. Again, the whole picture is one of the snowballing effect of interventions because, for instance, the IV apparatus and the fetal monitor constrict movement and restrict experimentation with different birth positions. And it is undeniable that the horizontal position is more convenient for the birth attendant—no bending down or squatting—than it is for the laboring woman. Surveys have shown that during delivery most women would prefer to stand, sit, or walk. There's also the belief that the lithotomy position keeps the women faceless, nonfunctioning above the waist, and thereby not engaged in active decision making—in short, it's a way for the practitioner, rather than the delivering woman, to control the birth.

What about the so-called primitive method—birth in a squatting position? Should you be interested in this and bring this up to your doctor, don't be surprised if he renders the opinion, a fairly common one in medical circles, that the modern Western woman does not have the posture to maintain such a position in labor for long periods without support. If this is his response, ask your doctor about the birth cushion. Developed in Britain, it's a U-shaped foam plastic cushion that supports the woman's thighs and has handles on both sides to help her push out the baby. Some British doctors say that it reduces the need for forceps deliveries and cuts time spent in the second stages of labor; however, a letter to the editor in the *British Medical Journal* (November 11, 1989) cautions "women who wish to give birth in the natural squatting position . . . to declare their intention early in pregnancy, so that they can prepare themselves with the help of physiotherapists."

And don't be afraid to turn the hospital routine on its ear and the birth position on its side, in a sitting position, on its back in a semisitting or propped position, or anyway you feel comfortable. Enlist your doctor's support in this matter beforehand.

Amniotomy

The deliberate breaking of the amniotic membranes (bag of waters) surrounding the baby, amniotomy is done to induce or start labor, to speed up labor already in progress, or to enable the internal fetal monitor to be attached to the baby's scalp. Here again, one intervention is creating the need or paving the way for another.

Shortening labor, one of the "accepted" rationales for amniotomy, is an attractive idea for many women (and their doctors). Why wait for the natural rupture of the bag of waters, which can occur anytime during labor or at birth? Roberto Caldeyro-Barcia, M.D., probably the leading name in research into the maternal and fetal effects of obstetric interference, specifically amniotomy, found that, at most, amniotomy reduces labor by thirty, maybe forty, minutes, *if at all*. Meanwhile, the natural watery barrier surrounding the fetus is gone, a factor that presents some risks to the baby as well as increases the chance of maternal postpartum infection.

Is it worth it? Certain conditions or problems may mandate

145

artificial rupturing. For instance, the doctor who suspects fetal distress may artificially rupture the membranes to see if the amniotic fluid is meconium-stained; the fluid, normally colorless, may appear greenish-brown and thus indicate the presence of meconium, actually a fetal bowel movement and a sign of possible fetal distress.

But childbirth procedures performed simply out of force of habit, or because they are part of standard hospital obstetric protocol or convenient timesavers are not sound medical practice. Ask what *your* doctor's practice is regarding amniotomy: when he does it and why. Of course, your birth plan should spell out the agreements you and your practitioner have come to, but, again, don't assume that these preferences will studiously be followed and that standard hospital routines will not be put in motion.

Electronic Fetal Monitoring

The debate over electronic fetal monitoring (EFM) is contentious—probably more so than for any other obstetric intervention since forceps delivery. An electronic fetal monitor is an instrument that measures uterine contractions *and* fetal heart rate during labor. Provided the device is working properly, the purpose is to monitor how the baby is tolerating labor, and there are two ways to do this, externally and internally. The external monitor, which generally uses ultrasound to pick up the heartbeat, has wide straps or belts that go around the woman's abdomen. With the internal monitor, a catheter is threaded through the vagina and an electrode placed on the baby's presenting part (usually the scalp) by means of metal clips or screws. It also requires that at least one strap be around the woman's abdomen and maybe another around her thigh. The readings from the internal monitor are reputedly more accurate than the external device, but critics of EFM cite newborn scalp infections as possible complications.

Electronic fetal monitoring was introduced in the 1960s and first used by American obstetricians in the early 1970s on the assumption that the monitoring device would alert the doctor to any problems that deprive the infant of oxygen—believed to be a cause of impaired neurological development—and that cause infant death. Thus alerted, the doctor could intervene in whatever presumably timely and appropriate fashion he deemed necessary. Reserved for high-risk pregnancies in its early applications, EFM, by the late 1970s, had become *routine practice in most hospitals, even though no scientific evidence of its safety and efficacy existed.* Even without controlled studies on risks and benefits, the entire scenario fit nicely into the traditional medical scheme of pregnancy and birth: a dangerous, risky time calling for medical interventions as the crises arise. While critics of the technology maintain that it often incorrectly indicates that a fetus is in distress and thereby leads to unnecessary cesarean sections, proponents contend that the device saves lives.

Today, EFM remains a widespread practice, with approximately three-quarters of births electronically monitored, but all is not well. Childbirth groups and consumers—the women who have been strapped, cinched, and immobilized by the technology, and their partners who, like the hospital staff in attendance, have been too immobilized and besotted by the bleeps and flashing lights of the monitor to attend to *the* business at hand—have long cried out against overreliance on this technology, and so have voices within the medical profession itself. This narrative from a letter written by a doctor to the editor of *Ob. Gyn. News* (July 15–31, 1989) addresses what many see as the root of the problem, medical education:

> The present-day obstetric resident has become mesmerized by the fetal monitor. I have no argument about its sensitivity, but its specificity is another matter. . . . On one occasion, I sent a patient to the hospital to be checked as to whether or not she was in labor. After a period of time, I called to find out her status. When I asked the on-duty resident if my patient was in labor, he said that he had not had time to place her on the monitor and, for that reason, he could not answer my question. . . . My final conclusion is that the current obstetric philosophy is embodied in the statement, "When in worry, fear, or doubt, grab a knife and cut it out."

Unlike the fetal monitoring of bygone or less technologically oriented times, which emphasized the practitioner-to-patient relationship and closeness, electronic gadgetry can too often serve as a crutch (as the doctor's letter quoted above illustrates), separate the birth attendants from the woman, and divert attention to the light show on the screen, rather than the human drama at hand. As William Ray Arney says in *Power and the Profession of Obstetrics* (Chicago: University of Chicago Press, 1982), "Monitoring changed the focus of interest of the profession from the mother to the fetus and thereby justified a wider array of interventions while, at the same time, it allowed the profession to make the claim that births were more natural and 'physiologic.'"

Two major studies, however, demonstrate that serious flaws underlie current medical thinking about EFM's value: namely, the idea that *routine* continuous electronic fetal monitoring greatly improves the health of newborns. In fact, an early study, published in the *New England Journal of Medicine* (September 4, 1986), of nearly thirty-five thousand births found that continuously monitoring fetal heartbeat in childbirth leads to slightly more cesarean-section deliveries, but does not produce healthier babies. Although continuous electronic monitoring is considered wise in high-risk pregnancies, the study concluded that "not all pregnancies, and particularly not those considered at low risk of perinatal complications, need continuous electronic fetal monitoring during labor."

The other, more recent study—a six-year joint American and Canadian project published in the *New England Journal of Medicine* (March 1, 1990)—is the first to suggest that the technology may actually do harm. The researchers found that electronic fetal monitoring appears to increase rather than reduce premature infants' risk of cerebral palsy, a group of brain disorders the technology was designed to prevent. The new study also supports eight previous studies that found no benefit from EFM when compared with careful, periodic monitoring using a specialized stethoscope called a fetoscope or using ultrasonography.

Ask your doctor what role electronic fetal monitoring—both periodic and continuous—plays in the hospital's protocol and the doctor's own standards of practice, and be prepared to call

148

attention to these two important studies, both appearing in a prestigious medical journal. If your doctor's response is "I do that for all my patients," ask why. Chances are he won't say that it's because of a fear of malpractice suits, yet the 1986 study and others have pinpointed just that as the rationale behind excessive medical intervention. Or if the doctor says that the hospital is too short-staffed and busy (a common complaint among medicos) to assign nurses to monitor periodically with stethoscope or ultrasonography, point out that it presumably takes staff to view the screen during EFM. Or find another hospital.

Finally, remind the doctor that the American College of Obstetricians and Gynecologists recommends that women with high-risk pregnancies (and premature birth would be one) have either continuous electronic fetal monitoring or intermittent checks with a stethoscope every fifteen minutes early on, and then every five minutes later. As for normal pregnancies, the group recommends only periodic monitoring (every thirty minutes early on and every fifteen minutes in later stages) by auscultation (listening with a stethoscope).

Induction and Augmentation of Labor

Induction is the artificial start of labor, before it begins spontaneously or naturally. Behind augmentation, or stimulation, of labor is the idea that labor is moving "too slowly" or "failing to progress" and so must be helped along. In either case, drugs are commonly used, administered intravenously, presumably so that the rate of flow and woman's response to the dosage can be carefully monitored. These interventions, both induction and augmentation, are best when used conservatively and reserved for absolute medical necessity—and, indeed, medically indicated obstetric drugs have saved the lives and health of many mothers and babies. Sally Inch, in *Birthrights*, for instance, mentions "some obstetrical conditions in which it may be hazardous for the pregnancy to continue to term" and in which induction of labor may be beneficial: essential maternal high blood pressure or kidney disease; preeclampsia, a toxic condition characterized by high blood pressure, edema, and protein in the urine; maternal diabetes; and Rhesus disease or isoimmunization (a blood incompatibility). Although not necessarily a risk factor, postmaturity (a prolonged pregnancy) is usually the most common reason given for induction, because of its association with placental insufficiency. In other words, the placenta has a limited life span and may not be able to sustain the baby properly in a too-long pregnancy.

But the practice around which all the controversy swirls is the *routine* or *elective* induction or stimulation of labor done as a matter of convenience for the doctor, the hospital, or even the mother, and not out of medical necessity. The authors of *Birth Trap: The Legal Low-down on High-Tech Obstetrics* (St. Louis, Missouri: Mosby, 1984) describe the sort of hospital timetable that gives the system its "assembly-line obstetrics" reputation:

> Hospitals emphasize speed and efficiency. Hospital space is limited and expensive. Every hospital service has its break-even point below which the service loses money, at which it pays for itself, and above which it makes a profit. Obstetrics is no exception. Delivery suites must reflect a high turnover rate to pay the mortgage on the first of the month and staff salaries every other Friday. From an economic point of view, hospitals cannot afford to allow women to labor at their own natural, unhurried pace.

The usual interventions employed are amniotomy (breaking the waters, see p. 145) to induce labor and intravenous administration of Pitocin to stimulate labor. What's the problem with artificial augmentation of labor? Just ask any woman who has been given Pitocin, the common synthetic version of the hormone oxytocin (itself naturally produced in the body of the laboring woman and instrumental in the progression of labor). Many, if not most, will report longer and stronger contractions and shorter intervals between contractions than they experienced in unstimulated labor. Thus, the stage is set for yet another intervention, in this case painkilling drugs for the relief of contractions of overwhelming intensity. As for possible adverse effects of elective stimulation of labor on the fetus, various reports relate how the strength and rapidity of contractions can decrease the ability of the fetus to restore its supply of oxygen between contractions. So the door swings open to yet another intervention, perhaps forceps delivery or a cesarean section.

Ask your doctor what his percentage of induced labors is and what the medical indications are. A response of more than 20 percent, says Elkins in *The Rights of the Pregnant Parent*, should certainly set off alarms, and actually, according to her own survey, "doctors who perform inductions *for medical indications only* induce less than 10 percent—some less than 5 percent."

Analgesics and Anesthetics

The use of obstetric drugs during labor and delivery is a controversial matter, with the staunchest critics citing the potentially harmful effects for both the mother and baby and the prevailing medical opinion being that, in small doses and at the right time, such drugs aid the woman and cause few or no adverse effects for the baby. At the heart of the controversy is the indisputable fact that almost all medications pass through the placenta and into the baby and, as the American Academy of Pediatrics says, no drug has been proved safe for the unborn child. A further indictment, at least in the minds of critics, is that "obstetric drugs used routinely for labor and delivery have not been approved for that purpose by the [Food and Drug Administration], and thus they assume the status of experimental drugs" (*The New Our Bodies, Ourselves* [New York: Simon & Schuster, 1984]). This means that you should be just as cautious during labor and delivery as during the prior nine months about the drugs and medications you take. The problem is that, unlike the stern admonitions about drug-taking most women get from their doctors during pregnancy, the majority of these same doctors routinely give or order analgesics (painkillers) and anesthetics.

Pain relief is the prevailing reason for giving most drugs during hospital birth—the stock medical rejoinder being "To make you as *comfortable* as possible"—and certainly there may

151

be sound medical grounds for doing so (just make sure your doctor spells out what they are far in advance of your labor and delivery). But too often it is the birth attendants' *perception* that you are in pain and in need of relief that cranks up the well-oiled machinery of hospital routine and obstetric interventionism. "A pharmaceutical feast" is how *Birth Trap* depicts the use of drugs in the traditional hospital delivery scenario:

> She is offered sedative-hypnotics for fear and apprehension, narcotics for labor pains, tranquilizers to augment the narcotics, amnesics to obliterate the memory of pain, narcotic antagonists to reduce the adverse side effects of narcotics on the baby, antiemetics to reduce the adverse side effects of narcotics, anesthetics for pain of delivery, vasoconstrictors to reduce the adverse effects of the anesthetics, antacids to reduce the adverse effects of the anesthetics, and more oxytocin to hurry expulsion of the placenta or, in the case of cesarean sections, more narcotics for pain as well as prophylactic antibiotics to head off the high probability of infection.

Admittedly, this is a worst-case scenario, but it is certainly true that over- and injudicious use of analgesics and anesthetics is detrimental to both mother and baby. Indeed, many of the most widely used analgesics can cause depression of the baby's central nervous system, which can appear as fetal distress on a fetal monitor. From there it's only a short slide into more obstetric interventions—cesarean section, to name a likely one.

Why, then, do doctors routinely administer obstetric pain-relief medications and anesthetics? Most commonly, Demerol (the generic name is meperidine) is the analgesic used during childbirth, either through an IV or by injection. A narcotic, Demerol is used to relax the woman, ease pain, and "help her rest during contractions," says *The Columbia University College of Physicians and Surgeons Complete Guide to Pregnancy*. But, like other drugs for obstetric pain relief, it can slow or prolong labor, or stop it entirely. Often in these instances the stock medical response is to administer labor-stimulating drugs, which may in turn increase pain and, thus, the need for more painkillers. Aside from the depressant effects the drugs can have on the baby, there is also the risk of starting the newborn on a merry-go-round of interventions. For the lethargic baby who is not breathing too well, it is not uncommon for the doctor to administer another drug to counteract or reverse the effects of the analgesic.

Skeptics of traditional medical practice cite the convenience and control that obstetric drugs offer doctors. As the authors of *Birth Trap* point out, "Drugged patients are usually quiet, compliant, and easily manipulated. . . . Drugs not only increase power over patients but also power over time. They contribute enormously to predictability, routinization, and convenience of birth events." Besides, where would the practice of obstetrical anesthesiology be without drugs in hospital births?

The use of local anesthesia entails numbing medication injected into specific tissue. Two forms of it are (1) pudendal block, usually given at the end of labor, which anesthetizes the vulva (external female organs), vagina, and muscles of the pelvic floor; and (2) paracervical block, which anesthetizes the lower uterus, cervix, and upper vagina, but which is being used less and less because the site of injection is too close to the fetal placenta.

Regional anesthesia, in the obstetric context, causes loss of sensation in the lower half of the body. Probably the most widely used form is the lumbar epidural, also known as *continuous* regional anesthesia because the anesthetic can be continuously readministered during delivery. Through a tiny catheter placed in the back—and often inserted even before the onset of labor as in the case of induction—the epidural is administered by injection into a hollow space in the spine. Some of the advantages touted are that it deadens pain without dulling mental faculties but only partially affects motor function; however, the woman needs coaching on when to push since she cannot feel contractions.

According to the procedure's critics, epidurals, although popular, are not without risks and potential iatrogenic mishaps, including accidental lumbar puncture, in which the needle is pushed too far; hypotension (sudden drop or lowering of mother's blood pressure—and possible subsequent lack of oxygen to the baby); and postdelivery complications such as numbness in the legs or difficulty walking. On the other hand, says Gerta Marx, M.D., a noted anesthesiologist at New York City's Einstein Medical College,

> When administered properly, epidurals carry a very low incidence of complications. And hypotension can be avoided if the procedure is managed properly. In my experience, OBs and midwives report very few complications, although sometimes general practitioners encounter some of these situations. The woman must be told to bear down when the epidural is given; then there are no complications.

In regional anesthesia, other interventions may or may not be necessary, including IV (for the administration of the anesthetic); amniotomy and/or labor-inducing drugs (to speed along labor that has been slowed or stopped by the drug); electronic fetal monitoring (to monitor the effects of the drug on the baby); or cesarean-section delivery.

Once used extensively but now replaced by the epidural as the "anesthesia of choice," the saddle block, or spinal, is another form of regional anesthesia. It anesthetizes from the stomach to the toes, totally stops labor and motor functions, and necessitates forceps or vacuum extraction delivery. According to Sheila Cohen, M.D., chair of the committee on obstetrics of the American Society of Anesthesiologists, a saddle block may be used on occasion to relieve pain during a forceps delivery. Aside from the possible undesirable aftereffects of any anesthesia, such as a headache, backache, or stiff neck, the spinal also carries more serious risks, especially if administered improperly: heart and lung failure, and even death, have resulted on occasion.

Clearly, given the risks, complications, and controversies surrounding these and other forms of obstetric drugs, you should discuss the entire matter with your doctor long before you are involved in your labor and delivery. Ask your doctor what percentage of his delivering women are given analgesics and/or anesthetics, in what forms, under what circumstances or conditions, and why. And remember, it is your childbirth experience—you have every right to call the shots, within the bounds of medical safety, of course, but you need a supportive practitioner and environment. Furthermore, if you feel you need them, you have the right to have medications. Just be sure you have discussed the relative risks and benefits with your doctor.

Forceps

Actually a surgical instrument, obstetric forceps are metal blades used to grasp the sides of the baby's head and help guide the baby through the birth canal in difficult deliveries. In general, forceps are employed when anesthesia or the position of the baby prevents the mother from pushing the baby out herself, when there is severe fetal distress, or when certain maternal conditions necessitate shortened labor and delivery.

The debate over forceps, however, has more to do with their use in uncomplicated deliveries, when there is no medical need to hurry the delivery, a use described as elective or prophylactic (preventive). Partly because of medical training and its emphasis on the doctor's importance in and control over labor and delivery, for some hospitals and doctors elective use of forceps is "the way it's done." They justify the procedure by saying, "It makes delivery easier." But even when done by a skilled practitioner, the procedure is not without dangers to the mother— lacerations, hemorrhage, and infection, to name a few—and it necessitates further intervention: namely, a painkilling drug and an episiotomy. Some of the risks for the baby are hemorrhage and damage to the head and/or brain, nerve damage, and bruising or disfigurement.

True, there are varying degrees of interventionism in forceps delivery. The terms *low*, *mid-*, and *high* refer to how far into the birth canal the forceps are inserted. While the majority of forceps deliveries are low, some doctors believe themselves skilled enough to perform safely a mid-forceps delivery, although today most experts agree that even in the best of hands, mid-forceps carries potentially serious problems and poses greater dangers to mother and baby than low forceps. And high forceps delivery is considered too risky to be done.

Rather than incur the risks associated with any form of

forceps delivery and in order to accomplish the same thing—prompt removal of the baby, whether for convenience or out of medical necessity—an increasing number of doctors are performing cesarean sections.

Another instrument for mechanical means of delivery is the vacuum extractor. Considered less risky and disfiguring than forceps, the procedure involves a small suction cup, which is placed on the baby's head, and the creation of a vacuum to draw out the baby. As with any other medical interference in the birth process, however, it can be improperly applied, and its success depends on the practitioner's skill and expertise.

In either of these approaches, the watchwords are speed and efficiency, the need for which is perceived primarily by hospital staff and birth attendants. Hence, you hear talk of "slow labor" or "failure to progress." While this certainly may be a true state of affairs, many times it results from earlier interventions that themselves inhibit labor.

Find out where your doctor stands in this debate—and remember our earlier caveat: if you do not discuss the issue and negotiate to prevent its use, you stand a chance of having this technology or procedure used on you, whether or not your labor is normal.

Episiotomy

An episiotomy is an incision made in a woman's perineal tissue—tissue that extends from the vagina to the anus—to enlarge the opening for birth, following which the incision is sewn up. The medical rationale behind the procedure? It aids the delivery, reduces compression of the baby's head (from battering against the perineal obstruction), and prevents tearing of the tissue, specifically third- and fourth-degree tears (to the anal sphincter and through the rectum).

So routine is the procedure (estimates run somewhere between 85 and 90 percent of births), and so pervasive, that many women believe—and doctors have told them—that without an episiotomy there would be severe, jagged tears and that the procedure is virtually mandatory for a woman's first delivery. Indeed, many women believe—and doctors have told them—that a surgical cut is preferable to a jagged tear. Underlying these opinions, too, is the belief that episiotomy prevents excessive stretching of the perineum and subsequent enlargement of the vagina and loss of muscle tone there. Without an episiotomy, so the argument goes, sexual satisfaction is reduced.

Critics of the procedure, however, assert that the benefits are iffy, except in certain cases of fetal distress, and that it creates just as many problems, and often more, than it is alleged to prevent, including postpartum pain and discomfort. And no evidence supports the various reasons doctors give for performing the surgery. In fact, research supports the contention that severe tears are not more frequent in deliveries without episiotomy, and that no other benefit has been proven for the *routine* use of episiotomy. A joint Johns Hopkins University and University of Hawaii study, published in the May 1989 *American Journal of Obstetrics and Gynecology*, concluded that episiotomy is "associated with a decrease in perineal lacerations of first- and second-degree, but a fourfold increase in the incidence of third-degree lacerations." And a major study some years back of more than twenty-one thousand deliveries, reported in the August 1985 *British Journal of Obstetrics and Gynecology*, lent further weight to earlier findings: namely, that episiotomy is needed in no more than one in every five deliveries.

Furthermore, detractors point out that episiotomy is the quintessence of circular illogic: lithotomy position for birth, preferred and popularized by obstetricians, actually creates the need for episiotomy, while at the same time episiotomy dictates the position because the procedure is easier to perform that way. Even stirrups, an apparatus favored by obstetricians, creates a tension in the perineum that may cause tears or lead to episiotomy. The perineal tissue normally stretches at the vaginal opening to allow the baby's head to be born—that is, if care is taken—but obstetricians just are not trained to do it any other way. True to their education and orientation, they stand ready to cut rather than employ tried-and-true midwifery techniques, such as changing the traditional hospital birth position to an upright, sitting, or squatting one; massaging the perineal tissue with oils and wet compresses; helping the delivering woman relax with breathing and other techniques; and coaching properly so that the baby can be eased out without damage to either the mother or the baby.

As with so many other critical issues, you will want to discuss this with your doctor as early as possible. Of course, realize that valid medical indications for episiotomy may arise at the time of imminent delivery. But at least you can begin the negotiating process and assert your wishes. Be sure to ask your doctor what indications—maternal exhaustion, baby size, and so on—he sees as necessitating episiotomy and what measures he takes to prevent the need for the surgery. In mulling over your choices, ask your doctor about the complications associated with the procedure, such as pain, bleeding, and infection.

Cesarean Section

Of all the issues you face as you prepare for childbirth, cesarean section (or c-section)—a surgical procedure in which the doctor cuts through the abdomen and uterus to remove the baby—is the most controversial: the hands-down winner if you are looking for the topic that raises the most eyebrows in a group of childbirth educators, sets the majority of tongues and chins wagging in a meeting of obstetricians, and appears regularly in medical journals, popular magazines, and newspapers nationwide. Ralph Nader's Public Citizen Health Research Group says that it is the number-one unnecessary surgery in the United States. Health policy analysts, renegade voices within the medical profession, and consumer groups call it a national epidemic. And just about every critic dubs it "the ultimate medical intervention in childbirth." Meanwhile, the practice is defended by many, if not most, medical professionals who see themselves ensuring safe deliveries and more perfect babies.

Today, one of four pregnant women in the United States will give birth by cesarean section—a rate higher than any other country in the world, according to the National Center for Health Statistics. (As mentioned earlier, Britain considers its 11 percent rate a crisis.) At one time, c-section was considered a last resort, an emergency lifesaving event for mother and baby—a less than 5 percent rate for a practitioner was a "hallmark of good obstetric practice," says a *Journal of the American Medical Association* (September 15, 1989) editorial. In 1970, the rate of cesarean births in this country stood at just 5.5 percent of all live births. But between 1970 and 1987, the rate skyrocketed to its present level—without a corresponding drop in the infant or maternal mortality rate—and researchers at the National Center for Health Statistics predict that without a change in obstetrical delivery trends, the rate of c-section could reach 40 percent by the year 2000.

While all regions of the country have seen sharp increases, the highest rates generally are in the Northeast and South and the lowest in the Midwest and West. Rates are lowest for hospitals with the fewest beds, and increase with the size of the hospital. Government hospitals have lower rates than nonprofit or proprietary (for-profit) hospitals, and women with private insurance are more likely to go under the knife than Medicaid-covered or uninsured women (*Statistical Bulletin*, October–December 1989).

Along with ire, questions have been raised. *Are women, their pregnancies, or their babies so different nowadays as to justify such a prodigious increase? Do differences in women and pregnancies from one section of the country to another explain regional variations in c-section rates? Is c-section so safe—indeed, so much safer than vaginal birth— and so preferable that the rates merely reflect the appropriateness of the medical decision to perform one? Or are there nonmedical factors at work here?*

Straightforward analyses of the trend to higher and higher rates have found four indications responsible for most cesarean deliveries:

- Previous cesarean section, the leading cause of cesareans. More than one-third are performed in the name of the dictum "Once a cesarean, always a cesarean."
- Breech presentation. Rather than the usual head-first presentation, the baby presents bottom-first ("frank breech") or feet-first ("footling breech").

- Dystocia (abnormal or difficult labor), the second leading cause of cesareans.
- Fetal distress (associated with increased use of electronic fetal monitoring).

Traditionally, c-section has been considered medically necessary and safer than vaginal birth in a number of high-risk situations, including

- multiple birth;
- delivery of a large infant (fetus/pelvis disproportion);
- delivery involving a woman with a serious condition or health problem such as infection; *abruptio placentae*, separation of the placenta from the uterine wall; or *placenta previa*, in which the placenta extends over the opening of the cervix;
- prolapse of the umbilical cord; and
- breech birth.

However, experts both within and outside the medical profession recount several widely held myths that they say have done more to drive up the numbers of c-sections than sound medical judgment.

Mortimer Rosen, M.D., chairman of Columbia University medical school's department of obstetrics and gynecology, has written one of the definitive books on this topic. In *The Cesarean Myth* (New York: Penguin Books, 1989), he sets forth, and subsequently refutes, three key misapprehensions concerning cesareans:

- *They are safe.* On the contrary, he says, as a form of major surgery, the emergency c-section poses a 400 percent higher risk of death to the mother than does vaginal birth, and elective cesarean (done for nonmedical reasons) a 200 percent higher risk. Not only is the recovery period longer and more difficult than with vaginal birth, but certain complications are nearly impossible to avoid: pain (often necessitating painkillers and their attendant problems); infection (the most common problem and one that requires further medication, antibiotic treatment); the aftereffects associated with anesthesia, such as bad headaches; and bleeding, sometimes excessive enough to require a transfusion (with attendant risks of its own).

• *They are absolutely necessary in a broad range of situations.* Along with others, Rosen says that actually the need for a c-section should be evaluated on a case-by-case basis because only a few broadly defined conditions or predicaments warrant the intervention, such as certain breech births and situations in which the placenta is attached in the wrong place. But clearly that cautionary approach is not in force in medical practice today. Instead, when doctors come across any uncertainty in the progress of labor or anything less than perfectly normal, many of them call for the operating room and the knife. With so many doctors racing to the operating room and hustling women into surgery, a lot of women are having *first* cesareans (and subsequently are in a flight pattern for repeats), even though the need may be vague or clinically unsubstantiated.

For example, cesarean delivery of the low- or very-low-birth-weight infant is a fairly standard obstetric practice, the idea being that a very small baby may not survive a vaginal delivery. The results of a five-year study reported in the *Journal of the American Medical Association* (September 15, 1989) belittle that idea. Analysis of birth and death certificates from Missouri, a state that is representative of the national experience in c-sections, between 1980 and 1984 revealed that c-sections don't alter survival chances of low-birth-weight infants. The study also concluded that there is little justification for the remarkable increase (from 24 to 44 percent) in c-sections for very small infants (1 to 3½ pounds).

• *They produce healthier, "better" babies.* Rosen echoes many other experts in the field who find no substantive evidence that c-sections are better for babies than are vaginal deliveries. "[The] recent dramatic rise in cesareans," he says, "has not reduced overall infant mortality rates or produced a generation of healthier babies." Even with the highest cesarean rate around, the United States nevertheless ranks twenty-second among nations in its infant mortality rate, according to the latest (1987) Centers for Disease Control calculations. And as major surgery, a c-section poses risks not only for the mother but also for the baby, including risk of iatrogenic, or doctor-

caused, conditions; respiratory distress; and carryover effects
from the drugs and anesthetics given the mother.

Shedding Light on "the Dark Side." Other, perhaps less in-
dulgent or kindly critics of cesareans who have looked deeper
into the heart of the beast say that myths do not tell the whole
story, that there are rampant nonmedical motivations at work
here. Herbert H. Keyser, M.D., in his book *Women Under the
Knife: A Gynecologist's Report on Hazardous Medicine* (Philadelphia: Stickley, 1984), calls these "the dark side of the increase [in cesareans]."

- *The Profit Motive.* Cesareans are more lucrative than normal
  vaginal deliveries. The doctor's fee is higher, the hospital stay
  is longer—nearly twice as long as vaginal deliveries, says a
  Journal of the American Medical Association (February 2,
  1990) article, with an average stay somewhere around four to
  five days, assuming no complications—and more hospital services and resources are required. In a 1989 survey of costs,
  the Health Insurance Association of America found that cesarean births cost two-thirds more than normal deliveries (the
  average cost for a vaginal delivery: $4,334), primarily because
  of higher hospital charges (*Modern Healthcare*, January 15,
  1990). With $5,133 the average hospital charge, and $2,053
  the average physician charge, a cesarean birth typically costs
  $7,186. (This stacks up against $2,111, the average cost of a
  one-day stay in a birthing center for a normal delivery—a figure, by the way, that includes professional fees. As for a mid-
  wife-assisted vaginal delivery, her average charge is $994.)
      Here is a different spin on the greed factor: family income,
  more than any medical risk factors, may determine how a
  woman will deliver, with the wealthiest women having a higher
  rate of c-sections. A University of California, Berkeley, study of
  nearly 246,000 childbearing women found nearly twice the rate
  of first-time cesareans among women whose family income
  topped $30,000 as among those earning less than $11,000
  (*New England Journal of Medicine*, July 27, 1989).

- *The Convenience Factor.* A typical scenario finds the obstetrician sitting around the hospital doctors' lounge or nurses'

station waiting for a woman's labor to run its course so that the doctor can "be there for her" in the minutes before birth. But what if her labor, as many other women's before her, takes longer than scheduled? If it is the beginning of the day, the doctor has patients to see during office hours, and at the end of the day—well, there are other commitments, possibly even a golf game. Even if the woman desires to labor a little longer, why wait to see whether there truly is a problem? Not only does inactivity waste the doctor's time, but it does not pay very well either. Given such economics, is it not easier for the doctor to consider possible fetal distress or possible dystocia and opt for a c-section?

Keyser says that "except for previously scheduled c-sections, which are usually done in the early morning, by far the greatest number are done immediately after office hours."

- *A Matter of Education and Training (or Lack Thereof)*. Obstetrical training emphasizes high-risk care and the extensive use of technology in labor and delivery. Doctors today receive very little training in normal deliveries and, with one in four births a cesarean, very little experience either. The skills, such as those required to turn around breech babies for vaginal deliveries, just are not there. A study of more than six thousand deliveries at a New York City hospital, reported in the July 1989 *American Journal of Obstetrics and Gynecology*, found some correlation between physician characteristics and the cesarean rate: namely, that older, more experienced doctors perform "significantly fewer cesarean sections for [difficult labor] and a higher percentage of forceps deliveries and breech [births]." But there seems to be encouraging news: a 1990 survey of physicians' practice habits by the American College of Obstetricians and Gynecologists found that, with respect to the area where the highest rate of cesareans has been (namely, in women who previously had cesarean deliveries), 98 percent of doctors under the age of forty encouraged vaginal delivery—versus 84 percent of doctors over age fifty-five. This is good news.

- *Entrenched Practice Patterns, Which Doctors Are Loath to Modify*. How else to explain the variation in c-section rates from practitioner to practitioner, hospital to hospital, and region to region? Practice habits, peer pressure, and other nonmedical factors seem to play a large role. Many doctors are reluctant to try tactics, for example, that were used successfully by midwives for centuries to help delivering women overcome problems in labor: changes in birth position, change in environment, walking, warm shower or bath, and breast and nipple stimulation.

Entrenched habits can be changed, however, A few basic rules and a prenatal review program are the key. This was the conclusion of a two-year study at a Chicago hospital that significantly reduced its c-section rate *without adverse effects on either the mothers or the infants*. The c-section rate there dropped from 17.5 percent in 1985 to 11.5 percent in 1987, as reported in the *New England Journal of Medicine* (December 8, 1988). The secret to the hospital's success?

- Second opinions by board-certified obstetricians were required for all cesareans, but no opinion could be obtained from the physician's associates in practice.
- Vaginal deliveries were preferred for all women who had previously undergone c-sections as well as for most breech presentations.
- Any diagnosis of fetal distress (obtained from monitoring the baby's heart rate) had to be confirmed by a blood sample from the fetus.
- As an indication for a cesarean, dystocia was accepted "only after no progress of labor was observed for more than two hours of regular uterine contractions."
- To ensure that doctors followed this program, a strict peer-review process was set up.

- *Defensive Medicine.* When asked why they perform cesareans, doctors say it is because they are afraid of being sued. Cesareans, so goes their thinking, are defensive medicine because, if the baby turns out less than perfect, the doctor is "covered" legally. But ask women who have had c-sections what rationales their doctors presented, and you find that most were told they and/or their babies were in distress. Nothing was mentioned about fear of litigation. Everything was couched in terms of medical necessity.

How Can You Avoid an Unnecessary Cesarean? Certain factors predispose a woman to cesarean surgery:

- If it is her first pregnancy
- If she is over thirty-five years old
- If she lives in a particular region of the country or has private health insurance
- If her birth practitioner is an obstetrician

Once you know these factors, you can evaluate your own particular situation and discuss with your doctor your likelihood of having a cesarean.

Also:

■ *Ask your doctor what his c-section rate is, as well as the hospital's.*

One expert quoted in a *Medical World News* (December 28, 1987) article suggests that 10 percent is appropriate, while others advocate figures ranging from 7.6 to 12 percent. Unfortunately, you may not get an answer to this question because, even in the midst of a national epidemic, many providers do not know these statistics. Doctors especially may not be keeping such records. In any case, ask early enough so that you can continue to shop around for the right doctor.

■ *Ask what the doctor's definition of and indications for dystocia ("abnormal labor") are.*

Dystocia, a leading reason for cesareans, has been called a "wastebasket" or catchall term. Research reported in the *Canadian Medical Association Journal* (March 1, 1990) found that the diagnoses of dystocia are so high "that one wonders whether the criteria used to define 'normal' adequately reflect the actual variations in labor patterns among women." Get a good sense of what your doctor means by "abnormal labor," and if he says "failure to progress," ask what the rush is—and recount the Chicago hospital's experience.

■ *Ask, in the event of legitimate dystocia, what methods your doctor would be willing to try as alternatives to a cesarean.*

Maybe just waiting for time to take its course will be enough. The doctor's pledge (preferably in the form of a signed birth plan) to allow you to try different birth positions, walk around, rest or sleep, or just wait shows a supportive provider willing to share the reins of control.

■ *Ask what your doctor's training and experience are in vaginal breech deliveries, vaginal births after previous cesareans, premature rupture of membranes, large baby, multiple births, and any other deviations from the norm.*

■ *Ask whether your doctor will accept a flat fee for delivery, whether it is vaginal or cesarean.*

Some doctors do have procedure-neutral fees for deliveries. This way, the economic incentive to perform a cesarean is eliminated. By the way, help here may be forthcoming from the insurance industry, which is striving to curb rising c-section rates. Blue Cross and Blue Shield plans in several states have begun to reduce payment for cesareans to discourage scalpel-toting doctors, and of course to save themselves millions of dollars a year.

Finally, should surgical intervention be found to be absolutely necessary—you, your partner, and your doctor have weighed the risks and benefits and are convinced—must you discard all your notions of, say, a family-centered birth and succumb to the "childbirth as medical event" system? Absolutely not, but in order to retain much of the control of your own childbirth here again you must lay the groundwork early. This means finding a doctor—*and* hospital *and* anesthesiologist—who acknowledges the potential negative effects, both emotional and physical, of a cesarean and recognizes the mother's need for support. Throughout the questioning process, remember—having a c-section is never something to feel guilty about. You haven't failed. But having an unnecessary c-section is both an insult to your integrity and a risk to you medically.

- Find out ahead of time what red tape you need to cut and whose signatures you need for your partner or advocate-friend to remain with you throughout the surgery and on into the recovery room. You may hear talk of infection risks and intrusive presences. Just reassure hospital staff that your partner or advocate will take all the infection-control precautions the operating room staff do and will be as unobtrusive as anyone can be in a usually already overcrowded scene such as an operating room.

- Find out what preoperative medications, anesthetic drugs, and postoperative analgesics are standard, as well as any adverse reactions and side effects associated with each. If there are options available, discuss with your doctor what they are and what would be best for you—that is, what would make you as comfortable but keep you as alert as possible.

- Assuming your partner or friend can help (and you and your baby are well), tell the powers-that-be that you want your baby to remain with you in the recovery room and your hospital room—to facilitate the critical early bonding too often missing in cesarean deliveries when babies are separated from their mothers.

- Find out whether the hospital's sibling visitation policy is responsive to your needs and desires. It is much more comforting for everyone in the family when siblings visit the newborn in your hospital room rather than stare at the baby through a glass partition.

- Ask how long the typical hospital stay following a c-section is. You may want to get out of the hospital as soon as it is medically feasible, depending on how you feel. A four-day, or even longer, stay is not uncommon, depending on whether or not there are complications.

VBAC: Vaginal Birth After a Cesarean

You Have a Say-so in This Decision . . . But Don't Wait to Be Asked

Most of the increase in the nation's c-section rate can be attributed to the long-standing practice of automatically delivering by cesarean if the mother has previously delivered a child that way. Despite decades of consumer battles for safer, natural births and despite general agreement among medical authorities to encourage a trial of labor after a cesarean, doctors and hospitals have been sluggish in their movement away from the outdated "Once a cesarean, always a cesarean" dictum. Even when the American College of Obstetricians and Gynecologists (ACOG) issued strong guidelines some years back stating that repeat cesarean deliveries should no longer be routine, many entrenched providers refused to budge.

Generally, the decision comes down to the incision—the *uterine* incision, that is, and not the type of incision and subsequent scar the woman has on her skin. Repeat c-sections are routinely performed to prevent rupturing of the uterine scar, but improved methods of cesarean incisions have reduced the risk of rupture during subsequent labor. And in actuality, says *The Columbia University College of Physicians and Surgeons Complete Guide to Pregnancy*, rarely does the uterus rupture completely, and when it does, most ruptures occur long before labor begins.

ACOG estimates that between 50 and 80 percent of women who have low transverse uterine incisions can deliver vaginally unless specific complications arise. But the group's guidelines still recommend against vaginal birth for women with the classical uterine incision, a high vertical incision rarely used these days. In the event of an obstetric emergency, ACOG guidelines also call for hospitals to be able to begin a cesarean within thirty minutes of a failed trial of labor instead of the former time of fifteen minutes. (Anesthesia must be available within the thirty-minute period rather than immediately.)

Even with these guidelines, acceptance of VBAC has been gradual. True, the VBAC rate has risen from 2 percent in 1970 to 10 percent in 1987, but a Metropolitan Life Insurance Company report says that is still far below what many experts believe to be medically possible (*National Underwriter*, January 22, 1990). Also in the report is the astonishing statistic that fewer than half of all hospitals *even offer* a trial of labor to women who have had previous c-sections—even though the success rate for a vaginal birth among women allowed a trial of labor is about 50 percent. Clearly, this suggests that VBAC rates are low because the option is infrequently of-
(continued)

fered, and not because of failure of trial of labor.

You can do a number of things to ensure that you get a trial of labor, if you wish to have a vaginal birth after a previous cesarean delivery:

• First, *don't wait* for your doctor to recommend it. Long before your due date, talk to your doctor and make sure he is up-to-date on the most current recommendations by the American College of Obstetricians and Gynecologists. The group continually revises its guidelines in an effort to lower the overall cesarean rate and encourage an attempt at labor and VBAC.

• Take advantage of groups providing support and information about VBAC, some of the more prominent of which follow:

Cesarean Prevention Movement
P.O. Box 152
University Station
Syracuse, New York 13210
Telephone: 1-315-424-1942

Cesarean/Support, Education and
  Concern, Inc. (C/SEC, Inc.)
10 Speen Street
Framingham, Massachusetts 01701
Telephone: 1-508-820-2760

International Childbirth Education
  Association
P.O. Box 20048
Minneapolis, Minnesota 55420
Telephone: 1-612-854-8660

Your Baby Is Born!

Now your life as mother and child begins—but there are some immediate postdelivery issues to be prepared for and more long-term matters to be aware of.

• *Parent Options at Birth.* The traditional sequence of events at birth goes something like this: baby arrives; the umbilical cord is clamped in two places, and the cord cut between the clamps by the doctor or nurse. Nanoseconds later a nurse puts the identification bracelet(s) on the baby, and whisks the child away to have eye medication administered and be placed in an infant warmer. This is the way it has always been done—in the delivery room, in the movies—but it's not necessarily the way it *must* be done. Many experts agree that the baby's father or other companion can cut the umbilical cord—in fact, also receive ("catch") the baby as it is being born—and that a delay in cutting the cord is a good thing. By waiting until the cord

169

has stopped pulsing and emptied of blood, "the baby's oxygen supply is not suddenly cut off, requiring that the baby take its first breath within seconds of birth . . . [and] a delayed cord clamping appears to aid the placenta in separating from the uterus more quickly," says Bean (*Methods of Childbirth*). And hers is not the only voice echoing these sentiments. After all, what's the rush? *You* have waited nine months, so why can't the doctor and the hospital wait five to ten minutes before they wheel in the next money-maker? Talk to your doctor.

Speaking of time, that's exactly what many new parents are telling their doctors that they want more of: time with their baby immediately postdelivery. The need for and benefits of bonding have been verified in various animal and human studies. If this is an important issue to you, tell your doctor to arrange for your baby to be left with you for some time after birth, instead of immediately separated and placed in the warming "box" across the room from you. (After all, positive identification, fingerprinting, and photographing are for criminals just before they're incarcerated, and not for babies.)

This excerpt from the book *Benefits and Hazards of the New Obstetrics*, edited by Tim Chard and Martin Richards (Philadelphia: Lippincott, 1977), says it all (about many things, and specifically about bonding)—show it to your doctor:

> When mothers are happy and active participants in childbirth, they are eager to pick up their babies immediately on delivery. If there is peace, quiet, and time, they touch, explore, and cuddle their newborn, and may put it to the breast. This is a period of heightened sensitivity in the mother during which she interacts with her baby and begins to form a special attachment to it. All of this appears to have long-lasting effects on parental attachment, and may ultimately affect the development of the child.

But unlike anesthesia, drugs, and IVS, bonding is not a reimbursable procedure, so be prepared to arrange this in advance and assert yourself. True, the climate today is more competitive, especially with birth centers catering more to the needs and wishes of parents, and some hospitals have come around. But there are plenty that remain stuck in the assembly-line childbirth methods of long ago.

● *Rooming-In.* Here, again, the relentless machinery of the hospital may threaten to override your desires. Many hospitals still routinely separate mothers and their babies. Off to central lockup goes the baby, and off to recovery and then her room goes the new mother. Wherever the baby goes, so should go a parent, say consumer advocates, and we agree. If a doctor (often the baby's own pediatrician, about whom we have more to say later) wants to do a complete physical examination of your baby in the first hours after birth, then ask to have it done in your or your partner's presence so that you can see what's going on and voice concerns and ask questions.

   Rooming-in policies, as we said before, vary from hospital to hospital, so be ready in the event of conflict between what you want and what the hospital wants to deliver. You may believe rooming-in means keeping your baby with you as much as you want and maybe as much as twenty-four hours a day. The hospital, on the other hand, may mean that your baby can stay with you all day but must return to the nursery at night. (Some hospitals' rooming-in policies are actually called modified rooming-in because babies stay with mothers only when mothers desire it, or only during mealtimes or other set intervals.) A rooming-in policy may or may not mean that fathers are welcome at any time; in some hospitals, fathers are expected to abide by the set visiting hours, in others fathers come and go . . . well, like family members in their own homes. (Now that's family-centered care!) Find out what the story is in the hospital where you intend to deliver. Document—in your birth plan, on the consent form, and, if necessary, on a sign posted on your door—that your baby is not to be taken away from you without your permission and that all baby-care activities are to be done at your bedside.

   There's a good chance that, as justification for separating you and your baby and limiting the time you spend together in your room, hospital staffers will talk about the "sterile hospital nursery environment" and the "germs" you and visitors bring to your room. The fact is that hospitals themselves are breeding grounds of infection, which even have a name of their own—nosocomial (medical lingo for hospital-originated) infections—so be the watchdog for your health and the health of your baby, whose immune system is especially vulnerable. Insist that everyone entering your room wash their hands, before they touch you, touch your baby, plump your pillow, take your temperature, shake your hand, whatever. (And, by the way, the risk of acquiring a nosocomial infection is another good reason to keep your baby close by your side—that way, you know if the nurses or aides have washed their hands first.) Talk to your doctor (and the baby's doctor, too) so that they can put their signatures to doctors' orders to that effect.

Go Home!

Call it reimbursement strategy, call it eagerness to get another paying customer in the bed, call it medically wise—but doctors and hospitals are discharging new mothers and their babies sooner than in times past when women stayed for nearly a week. Nowadays, women with normal, vaginal deliveries without complications go home in about two days or even less; in freestanding birthing centers, they go home within twelve to twenty-four hours. Make arrangements with your doctor and the hospital if you wish to go home sooner.

But bear in mind that a number of factors come into play here: How do you feel? Do you have other children at home? Do you have household help? Will your insurance company pay for an extra day, should you decide you need one? And if not, can you manage the costs yourself? You have to balance these with the hazards of any hospital stay: the risk of you or your baby acquiring a nosocomial infection; the less-than-endearing sounds and other interruptions so much a part of hospital routine—those squeaky carts that go by your door in the night, not to mention talkative hospital staffers that go by night and day—and everything else that can interfere with your recovery and with getting to know your baby.

Tips on Your Departure

Plan ahead as best you can for your leave-taking:

- Time your exit to save yourself some money. If hospital room rates are calculated from noon to noon, then leave before noon.

our Baby's Doctor

is sensible to have your baby's octor—family practitioner, pediatrician, or nonphysician specialist uch as a pediatric nurse practitioner, whatever your preference s—chosen *before* your due date. Don't wait until the last minute. Although we have placed this section ere at the end of the journey, because your and your baby's relationship with this practitioner actually egins when your relationship with our birth practitioner (at least for this particular pregnancy) is ending, you should have seen your baby's doctor for a prenatal consultation (usually in the last trimester).

Ask: "What do you charge for hospital consultations and office visits?" "Do you set aside time every day for phone consultations with parents? What do you charge for these?" "How long is the typical office appointment?" "How often do you want to see the baby in the first year? Second?" "Do you have a split waiting room so that sick children stay away from well children?"

More to the issue in this book, however: during the prenatal visit you can arrange for the doctor to attend the actual birth, if that is your desire, even should the delivery be uncomplicated and your baby normal and healthy. Whether the baby's doctor is present during and after delivery has a lot to do with the obstetrician (or other birth practitioner) and the hospital's protocol.

True, certain conditions that are known prior to delivery (fetal prematurity or postmaturity, multiple birth, maternal diseases such as toxemia, and the like) may require that the baby's doctor be right there, ready to assist should the need for neonatal intensive care or whatever arise. Otherwise, if you wish for the baby's doctor to attend the birth, talk to your doctor *and* the baby's doctor about it.

Should your baby be a boy, another postpartum issue that needs advance discussion is the question of circumcision, which usually is performed by the obstetrician a day or so after birth (and requires written consent of the mother). As a matter of fact, circumcision is the only male surgery done by the ob-gyn, the sole exception to the rule that obstetric responsibility for the baby ends at the cutting of the umbilical cord.

The American College of Obstetricians and Gynecologists contends there is no medical need for routine circumcision and that the parental decision to have or to not have the surgery performed is a personal one—requiring knowledge and forethought. Discuss the pros and cons with your doctor. Also be aware that circumcision is no longer offered on a routine basis at some hospitals and that an increasing number of health insurance plans do not cover routine circumcision.

Another topic that deserves

173

some thought and planning prior to the day of delivery is breast-feeding. Make it one of the major points of discussion with the prospective baby doctor, but realize, too, that infant-formula companies exert no small amount of influence with pediatricians and other baby doctors. If you are going to call the shots in the hospital concerning the nourishment your baby receives (for instance, breast milk only), where the baby receives it (if you are pressing for rooming-in during mealtimes), and what your baby is not fed (such as bottle-fed supplements in the nursery), then you need the support of your doctor and the baby's doctor, too. Lay the groundwork with both early. For information on breast-feeding, call the local chapter of La Leche League or contact the national office: La Leche League International, 9616 Minneapolis Avenue, Franklin Park, Illinois 60131; telephone 1-708-455-7730.

Why leave at 1:00 P.M. when it's cheaper to leave at 11 A.M., and you have been ready since bright and early that morning? Doctors, for all the admitting and discharging they do, are often fuzzy on the fine points such as when another day's room charge kicks in, so take it upon yourself to remind her of these details and lobby for an early exit.

● Ask about the post-hospital continuation of your care when your doctor comes around to discharge you. (If the doctor isn't there when you are ready to leave, or didn't let you know in person that you could go home, refuse to pay the doctor's discharge fee.) Ask when you should see her back in the office for a checkup. (Most doctors recommend that the first postpartum checkup take place in four to six weeks, and some as early as three weeks or as late as eight.) How much follow-up care is a part of the fee already charged you for her maternity care services? When can you resume a regular diet, exercise regimen, sex life, and so on? What can you do to speed your recovery—especially if you have had an episiotomy or a cesarean delivery—and forestall a relapse or infection? What signs should you watch for that could indicate trouble? Usually, the postpartum examination concludes the pregnancy, although hormonal and some physical changes continue to occur as the woman's body readjusts. Ask your doctor what to expect and also what is outside of the norm and may necessitate a phone call.

- If you haven't already discussed the need for further care, specifically a "baby nurse" for that first week or so of adjustment at home, do so now if you so desire. An appropriate hospital staff person should be able to suggest some names. Or you can contact local nursing agencies or even ask friends who have used baby nurses.

- Ask for an itemized bill from the hospital. You will want to review your bill with some care (not right there at the cashier's desk but later, at home, when you have time) to pick out any overcharges and dispute them. Some years ago Atlanta-based Equifax Services, Inc., audited thousands of hospital bills and found that 96.9 percent of them contained charges for services that were never performed. If you did not buy the traditional labor-and-delivery package, with its many routine procedures—IV, analgesic and anesthetic drugs, episiotomy, and so on—you should be doubly diligent about checking the charges. This is important even if you have health insurance. You are working to keep your bill down, and if everybody did that the rates wouldn't go up as much or as fast as they do. (Of course, if you don't have insurance, or have only minimal coverage, it is vital to your financial interest that you pore over your bill.) If necessary, take the bill with you when you see your doctor on the follow-up visit. She may be able to help decode any cryptic charges.

Future Pregnancies

It may be unseemly to bring up the subject of your next pregnancy. But it is not necessarily unrealistic or impractical. Family planning, after all, is not only for families who want a certain number of children but also for those who want their children spaced a certain number of years apart. Birth control needs change throughout your life—and especially so after you have had a baby. Sometimes a new mother's menstrual cycle takes a while to regulate itself. And while breast-feeding to a certain extent inhibits ovulation, this is not an absolute certainty and so should not be relied on. On the other hand, not every contraceptive method is open to the new mother—oral contraceptives are out if you are breast-feeding, and a diaphragm cannot be fitted immediately after childbirth.

Talk to your doctor about this no later than your first postpartum checkup. Also see your local telephone book for the Planned Parenthood affiliate/clinic nearest you, or contact the national office: Planned Parenthood, 810 Seventh Avenue, New York, New York 10019; telephone 1-212-541-7800.

Epilogue

There you have it. We have tried to present everything you need to know or ask in order to make sure that you have the pregnancy and childbirth that *you* want, and that you have it *your* way. Medical intervention often is critical, it's true, but routine medical practices should not, as they too often do, dictate in areas that are the woman's natural jurisdiction.

Now you're prepared and you're empowered. The process of regaining what should be yours naturally—the decision-making power over your body and your health—may not be easy. And you may bump up against more than a few obstacles. Just remember that you have choices, and armed with the information in this guide, you have the tools to make wise decisions.

Take this book to the obstetrician with you, and have a happy and healthy pregnancy.

Appendix A

Abruptio placentae   Premature separation of the placenta from the uterine wall.

Alpha fetoprotein (AFP)   Protein produced by the fetal liver and passed into the mother's blood via the placenta.

Amniocentesis   Extraction of a small amount of amniotic fluid in order to test for genetic and other disorders in the fetus.

Amniotic fluid   Watery fluid within the amniotic sac, which surrounds the fetus during pregnancy.

Amniotomy   Deliberate breaking of the amniotic membranes (bag of waters) surrounding the baby.

Antepartum hemorrhage   Heavy vaginal bleeding in the third trimester.

Artificial insemination by donor (AID)   Placement of donor semen into a woman's reproductive tract for purposes of conception.

Artificial insemination by husband (AIH)   Placement of the husband's semen into the wife's reproductive tract for purposes of conception.

Basal temperature   The body's lowest temperature in the course of a day.

Braxton-Hicks contractions   Mild, irregular contractions of the uterus; often called false labor or practice labor because they result in little or no labor development.

Breech presentation   Rather than a baby's usual head-first presentation, presentation of another part—bottom-first ("frank breech") or feet-first ("footling breech"), for example.

Centimeters   Measurement used to determine the opening, or dilation, of the cervix.

Cephalopelvic disproportion (CPD)   Condition in which the head or presenting part of the fetus cannot engage or pass through the mother's pelvis.

Cerclage   Surgical closing of the cervix.

Cervical incompetence   Abnormality of the cervix that prevents it from keeping the fetus securely within the womb.

Cesarean section (c-section)   Surgical operation in which the doctor cuts through the abdomen and uterus to remove the baby.

Chorionic villus sampling (CVS)   Extraction and examination of a small fragment of the early placenta to detect genetic abnormalities in the fetus.

Cordocentesis (also called **percutaneous umbilical cord sampling, or PUBS**)   Method of sampling fetal blood by inserting (with ultrasound guidance) a needle through the uterine wall and into the umbilical cord; used to detect severe genetic blood disorders.

Crowning   Presentation of the largest part of the baby's head, making it visible at the opening of the vagina.

Diethylstilbestrol (DES)   Synthetic estrogen hormone once used to prevent miscarriages.

Dilation (also called **dilatation**)   Enlargement of the opening of the cervix.

Dilation and curettage (D&C)   Artificial opening of the cervix and removal of the uterine contents.

Down syndrome (also called **Trisomy 21**)   Congenital abnormality with both mental and physical effects.

Dystocia   Abnormal or difficult labor.

Eclampsia   Severe form of toxemia characterized by convulsions and coma (in addition to the usual symptoms of preeclampsia).

Ectopic pregnancy   Pregnancy in which the fertilized egg does not complete its descent but begins to develop outside the uterus, usually in one of the fallopian tubes (hence the term *tubal pregnancy*); occasionally, the fertilized egg may start to grow in the mother's abdominal cavity or on the ovary.

Edema   Swelling of body tissue due to a buildup of fluid.

Effacement   Thinning out (by shortening and flattening) of the cervix.

Electronic fetal monitor   Instrument that measures uterine contractions and fetal heart rate during labor. The monitor may be external or internal.

Embryo transfer   Fertility enhancement procedure in which a man's sperm are used to fertilize the egg of a donor via artificial insemination.

Endometrial biopsy Extraction of a small piece of tissue from the uterus for examination.

Endometriosis Gynecological disease in which endometrial tissue, normally found in the uterus, grows outside the uterus.

Engagement Lodging of a baby's presenting part firmly in the pelvis; also called lightening or dropping.

Epidural anesthesia Type of anesthesia and standard method of relieving pain during labor; a local anesthetic is injected into the epidural space surrounding the spinal cord, producing numbness from the waist down.

Episiotomy Incision made in a woman's perineal tissue (between the vagina and the anus) to enlarge the opening for birth.

Fetoscope Specialized stethoscope used to listen to fetal heart tones during pregnancy and labor.

Fetoscopy Visual examination of the fetus by means of a thin, periscopelike instrument that is directed through a small abdominal incision and into the amniotic sac.

Forceps Surgical instrument; metal blades used to grasp the sides of the baby's head and help guide the baby through the birth canal in difficult deliveries.

Gamete intrafallopian transfer (GIFT) Method of conception that involves removing eggs from a woman's ovary, combining them with sperm, and placing the mixture directly in the fallopian tube for fertilization to occur.

Gestational diabetes Special short-term form of diabetes that can develop in a normally nondiabetic woman during pregnancy.

Gestational hypertension Hypertension, or high blood pressure, that may develop for the first time after week 20 of pregnancy.

Gravida Pregnant woman.

Human chorionic gonadotropin (HCG) Hormone secreted by the placental tissue after implantation in the uterine wall; the substance sought in pregnancy tests.

Hysterosalpingogram X-ray picture of the uterus, fallopian tubes, and ovaries.

Hysteroscopy Visual examination of the uterus with an endoscope inserted through the vagina and the cervix.

Induction Artificial starting of labor, usually with the hormone Pitocin.

Infertility Inability to reproduce.

Intrapartum hemorrhage Heavy bleeding during labor.

Intrauterine death Death of a baby in the uterus after week 20.

Intrauterine growth retardation Failure of a fetus to grow in the uterus.

In vitro fertilization (IVF)   Method of conception in which eggs are retrieved from the ovary just prior to ovulation, combined with sperm, and fertilized outside the woman's body; then the fertilized eggs are returned to the uterus.

IV   Abbreviation for *intravenous*.

Laparoscopy   Visual examination of a woman's abdominal and pelvic cavity with a telescopic instrument inserted through a small abdominal incision.

Lithotomy   Conventional (supine) position for giving birth; the woman lies flat on her back with her knees bent and legs spread wide apart with stirrups.

Meconium   Greenish-brown substance that fills the fetal intestine and is usually discharged right after birth.

Miscarriage   Lay term for spontaneous abortion.

Mucus plug   Bloody plug that seals off the cervix during pregnancy.

Multigravida   Woman pregnant for the second or subsequent time.

Neural tube defects   Birth defects caused by faulty formation of the spinal cord during gestation.

Oxytocin   Pituitary hormone secreted during childbirth for the stimulation of uterine contractions and milk secretion; a synthetic form often administered to induce or hasten labor.

Paracervical block   Type of anesthesia that numbs the lower uterus, cervix, and upper vagina.

Pelvic floor muscles   Muscles surrounding the urethra, vagina, and rectum.

Pelvic inflammatory disease (PID)   Infection of one or more of the internal female sex organs often resulting from bacterial forms of sexually transmitted diseases.

Pergonal   Trade name for human menopausal gonadotropin, or HMG.

Perineum   Area between the anus and the genitals.

Placenta   Organ that nourishes the baby in the uterus from conception until birth.

Placenta previa   Placenta that is abnormally low in the womb and that either partially or completely covers the opening of the cervix.

Postcoital test   Examination of the woman's vaginal and cervical mucus shortly after intercourse to determine whether it and the sperm are compatible.

Postmaturity   Prolongation of pregnancy beyond week 42.

Postpartum hemorrhage   Heavy bleeding after delivery.

Preeclampsia   Toxic condition of pregnancy characterized by high blood pressure, edema, and protein in the urine.

181

Premature rupture of membranes Leakage of amniotic fluid before labor has begun.

Prematurity Birth of a baby about three weeks or more before the estimated date of delivery.

Prepping Shave (of the pubic area), enema, and intravenous feeding.

Presenting part First part of the baby to be born.

Preterm, or **premature, labor** Labor that begins before the due date, sometimes long before.

Primigravida Woman pregnant for the first time.

Prolapse of the umbilical cord Condition in which the umbilical cord falls below or in front of the baby's presenting part.

Pudendal block Type of anesthesia that numbs the vulva (external female organs), vagina, and muscles of the pelvic floor.

Quickening A baby's first movements in the uterus as noticed by the mother.

Semen analysis (or **semenalysis**) Series of tests carried out on one sample to determine sperm levels and motility ability.

Spontaneous abortion Miscarriage.

Spotting Loss of small amounts of blood from the vagina.

Surrogacy Fertility enhancement method in which a couple enters a contract with a woman who agrees to become pregnant via artificial insemination with the husband's sperm, and carry the pregnancy to term. After the baby is born, the man who provided the sperm is the legal father and the surrogate mother allows the father's wife to adopt the baby.

Teratogens Toxins that can cross the placenta and damage a developing fetus, causing birth defects or even fetal death.

Toxemia of pregnancy Another term for eclampsia or preeclampsia.

Toxoplasmosis Disease transmitted from animals, especially cats, to humans, which if during pregnancy can cause birth defects or fetal death.

Transverse lie Presentation of a baby's shoulder or side.

Ultrasound Sound waves of very high frequency used for diagnostic purposes. The resulting echoes are translated into pictures on a television monitor; the image itself is called a sonogram.

Vacuum extractor Instrument used for mechanical means of delivery. The procedure involves a small suction cup, which is placed on the baby's head, and the creation of a vacuum to draw out the baby.

Varicocele Varicose or swollen vein in the spermatic cord.

Vertex presentation Presentation of a baby's head.

Zygote intrafallopian transfer (ZIFT) Method of conception in which eggs are retrieved from a woman's ovary, combined with sperm, and fertilized outside the woman's body. After fertilization, the embryo is placed in the fallopian tube about eighteen hours later.

Appendix B

—————— *Licensing Boards (M.D.)*

Alabama Medical Licensure
  Commission
  P.O. Box 887
  Montgomery, AL 36101
  Telephone: 1-205-261-4116

Alaska Department of Commerce
  and Economic Development
  State Medical Board
  P.O. Box D-LIC
  Juneau, AK 99811
  Telephone: 1-907-465-2541

Arizona Board of Medical
  Examiners
  2001 W. Camelback Road
  Suite 300
  Phoenix, AZ 85015
  Telephone: 1-602-255-3751

Arkansas Board of Medical
  Examiners
  P.O. Box 102
  Harrisburg, AR 72432
  Telephone: 1-501-578-2448

California Board of Medical
  Quality Assurance
  1430 Howe Avenue
  Sacramento, CA 95825
  Telephone: 1-916-920-6393

Colorado Board of Medical
  Examiners
  1525 Sherman Street, #132
  Denver, CO 80203
  Telephone: 1-303-866-2468

Connecticut Board of Medical
  Examiners
  150 Washington Street
  Hartford, CT 06106
  Telephone: 1-203-566-1035

Delaware Board of Medical
  Practice
  Margaret O'Neill Building
  2nd Floor
  Dover, DE 19903
  Telephone: 1-302-736-4522

District of Columbia
  Occupational and Professional
  Licensing Division
  614 H Street, N.W.
  Room 904
  Washington, DC 20001
  Telephone: 1-202-727-7480

Florida Board of Medical
  Examiners
  1940 N. Monroe Street
  Tallahassee, FL 32399-0750
  Telephone: 1-904-488-0595

Georgia Composite State Board of Medical Examiners
166 Pryor Street, S.W.
Atlanta, GA 30303
Telephone: 1-404-656-3913

Hawaii Board of Medical Examiners
P.O. Box 3469
Honolulu, HI 96801
Telephone: 1-808-548-4100

Idaho State Board of Medicine
500 S. 10th Street
Suite 103
Boise, ID 83720
Telephone: 1-208-334-2822

Illinois Department of Registration and Education
320 W. Washington Street
Springfield, IL 62786
Telephone: 1-217-785-0800

Indiana Consumer Protection Division
219 State House
Indianapolis, IN 46204
Telephone: 1-317-232-6330

Iowa State Board of Medical Examiners
Executive Hills West
1209 E. Court Avenue
Des Moines, IA 50319
Telephone: 1-515-281-5171

Kansas State Board of Healing Arts
900 S.W. Jackson
Suite 553
Topeka, KS 66612
Telephone: 1-913-296-7413

Kentucky Board of Medical Licensure
400 Sherburn Lane
Suite 222
Louisville, KY 40207
Telephone: 1-502-896-1516

Louisiana State Board of Medical Examiners
830 Union Street
Suite 100
New Orleans, LA 70112
Telephone: 1-504-524-6763

Maine Board of Registration in Medicine
State House, Station #137
Augusta, ME 04333
Telephone: 1-207-289-3601

Maryland Physician Quality Assurance
P.O. Box 2571
Baltimore, MD 21215-0095
Telephone: 1-301-764-4777

Massachusetts Board of Registration in Medicine
10 West Street
Boston, MA 02111
Telephone: 1-617-727-3086

Michigan Board of Medicine
P.O. Box 30192
Lansing, MI 48909
Telephone: 1-517-373-1870

Minnesota State Board of Medical Examiners
2700 University Avenue West
Room 106
St. Paul, MN 55114
Telephone: 1-612-642-0538

Mississippi State Board of Medical Licensure
2688-D Insurance Center Drive
Jackson, MS 39216
Telephone: 1-601-354-6645

Missouri State Board of Registration for the Healing Arts
P.O. Box 4
Jefferson City, MO 65102
Telephone: 1-314-751-2334, Ext. 151

Montana Board of Medical
  Examiners
  1424 9th Avenue
  Helena, MT 59620
  Telephone: 1-406-444-4284

Nebraska Board of Medical
  Examiners
  301 Centennial Mall South
  Box 95007
  Lincoln, NE 68509
  Telephone: 1-402-471-2115

Nevada State Board of Medical
  Examiners
  P.O. Box 7238
  Reno, NV 89510
  Telephone: 1-702-329-2559

New Hampshire Board of
  Registration in Medicine
  Health and Welfare Building
  6 Hazen Drive
  Concord, NH 03301
  Telephone: 1-603-271-1203

New Jersey State Board of Medical
  Examiners
  28 W. State Street
  Trenton, NJ 08608
  Telephone: 1-609-292-4843

New Mexico Board of Medical
  Examiners
  P.O. Box 20001
  Santa Fe, NM 87504
  Telephone: 1-505-827-9933

New York State Department of
  Health
  Office of Professional Medical
  Conduct
  Empire State Plaza
  Tower Building
  Albany, NY 12237
  Telephone: 1-518-474-8357

North Carolina Board of Medical
  Examiners
  P.O. Box 26808
  Raleigh, NC 27611
  Telephone: 1-919-876-3885

North Dakota State Board of
  Medical Examiners
  City Center Plaza, Suite C-10
  418 E. Broadway Avenue
  Bismarck, ND 58501
  Telephone: 1-701-223-9485

Ohio State Medical Board
  77 S. High Street
  17th Floor
  Columbus, OH 43215
  Telephone: 1-614-466-3938

Oklahoma State Board of Medical
  Examiners
  5104 N. Francis, Suite C
  Oklahoma City, OK 73118
  Telephone: 1-405-848-6841

Oregon State Board of Medical
  Examiners
  1500 S.W. 1st Avenue
  Room 620
  Portland, OR 97201
  Telephone: 1-503-229-5770

Pennsylvania State Board of
  Medical Education and Licensing
  P.O. Box 2649
  Harrisburg, PA 17105
  Telephone: 1-717-787-2381

Puerto Rico Board of Medical
  Examiners
  Call Box 10200
  Santurce, PR 00908
  Telephone: 1-809-725-7903

Rhode Island Division of
  Professional Regulation
  3 Capitol Hill
  Providence, RI 02908
  Telephone: 1-401-277-2827

South Carolina State Board of
  Medical Examiners
  1220 Pickins Street
  Columbia, SC 29201
  Telephone: 1-803-734-8901

South Dakota State Board of
  Medical and Osteopathic
  Examiners
  1323 S. Minnesota Avenue
  Sioux Falls, SD 57105
  Telephone: 1-605-336-1965

Tennessee Board of Medical
  Examiners
283 Plus Park Boulevard
Nashville, TN 37217
Telephone: 1-615-367-6231

Texas Board of Medical Examiners
P.O. Box 13562
Capitol Station
Austin, TX 78711
Telephone: 1-512-452-1078

Utah Department of Commerce
Medical Licensing
160 East 300 South
P.O. Box 45802
4th Floor
Salt Lake City, UT 84145
Telephone: 1-801-530-6628

Vermont Board of Medical Practice
Secretary of State's Office
Pavilion Office Building
Montpelier, VT 05602
Telephone: 1-802-828-2673

Virgin Islands Department of
  Health
Attn: Licensure
St. Thomas Hospital
St. Thomas, VI 00801
Telephone: 1-809-774-0117

Virginia State Board of Medicine
1601 Rolling Hills Drive
Richmond, VA 23229
Telephone: 1-804-662-9908

Washington State Medical Boards
Division of Professional Licensing
P.O. Box 9012
Olympia, WA 98504
Telephone: 1-206-753-2205

West Virginia Board of Medicine
101 Dee Drive
Charleston, WV 25311
Telephone: 1-304-348-2921

Wisconsin Medical Examining
  Board
1400 E. Washington Avenue
P.O. Box 8935
Madison, WI 53708-8935
Telephone: 1-608-266-2811

Wyoming Board of Medical
  Examiners
Barrett Building, 3d Floor
Cheyenne, WY 82002
Telephone: 1-307-777-6463

187

Appendix C

Alabama Medical Licensure
  Commission
P.O. Box 887
Montgomery, AL 36101
Telephone: 1-205-261-4153

Alaska Osteopathic Medical Board
  Department of Commerce and
    Economic Development
  Division of Occupational
    Licensing
  P.O. Box D
  Juneau, AK 99811
  Telephone: 1-907-465-2541

Arizona Osteopathic Examiners in
  Medicine and Surgery
1830 West Colter Street
Suite 104
Phoenix, AZ 85015
Telephone: 1-602-255-1747

Arkansas Board of Medical
  Examiners
P.O. Box 102
Harrisburg, AR 72432
Telephone: 1-501-578-2448

California Board of Osteopathic
  Examiners
921 11th Street
Suite 1201
Sacramento, CA 95814
Telephone: 1-916-322-4306

Colorado Board of Medical
  Examiners
1525 Sherman Street
Denver, CO 80203
Telephone: 1-303-866-2468

Connecticut Osteopathic Medical
  Board
Department of Health Services
Division of Medical Quality
  Assurance
79 Elm Street
Hartford, CT 06106
Telephone: 1-203-566-1039

Delaware Board of Medical
  Practice
Margaret O'Neill Building
P.O. Box 1401
Dover, DE 19903
Telephone: 1-302-736-4522

District of Columbia Commission on Licensure to Practice the Healing Art
605 G Street, N.W.
Washington, DC 20001
Telephone: 1-202-727-5365

Florida Board of Osteopathic Medical Examiners
1940 N. Monroe Street
Tallahassee, FL 32399-0775
Telephone: 1-904-488-7546

Georgia Composite State Board of Medical Examiners
166 Pryor Street, S.W.
Atlanta, GA 30303
Telephone: 1-404-656-3913

Hawaii Board of Osteopathic Examiners
P.O. Box 3469
Honolulu, HI 96801
Telephone: 1-808-548-3952

Idaho State Board of Medicine
State House
Boise, ID 83720
Telephone: 1-208-334-2822

Illinois Department of Professional Regulation
320 West Washington
3rd Floor
Springfield, IL 62786
Telephone: 1-217-782-0458

Indiana Medical Licensing Board
1 American Square
Suite 1020
Box 82067
Indianapolis, IN 46282
Telephone: 1-317-232-2960

Iowa State Board of Medical Examiner
Executive Hills West
1209 E. Court Avenue
Des Moines, IA 50319
Telephone: 1-515-281-5171

Kansas Board of Healing Arts
900 S.W. Jackson
Suite 553
Topeka, KS 66612
Telephone: 1-913-296-7413

Kentucky Board of Medical Licensure
400 Sherburn Lane
Suite 222
Louisville, KY 40207
Telephone: 1-502-896-1516

Louisiana State Board of Medical Examiners
830 Union Street
New Orleans, LA 70112
Telephone: 1-504-524-6763

Maine Board of Osteopathic Examination and Registration
State House Station 142
Augusta, ME 04333
Telephone: 1-207-289-2480

Maryland Physician Quality Assurance
4201 Patterson Avenue
P.O. Box 2571
Baltimore, MD 21215-0002
Telephone: 1-301-764-4777

Massachusetts Board of Registration in Medicine
10 West Street
Boston, MA 02111
Telephone: 1-617-727-3086

Michigan Board of Osteopathic Medicine and Surgery
P.O. Box 30018
Lansing, MI 48909
Telephone: 1-517-373-6650

Minnesota State Board of Medical Examiners
2700 University Avenue, W.
Suite 106
St. Paul, MN 55114-1080
Telephone: 1-612-642-0538

Mississippi State Board of Medical Licensure
2688-D Insurance Center Drive
Jackson, MS 39216
Telephone: 1-601-354-6645

Missouri Board of Registration for the Healing Arts
P.O. Box 4
Jefferson City, MO 65102
Telephone: 1-314-751-2334

189

Montana Board of Medical
Examiners
1424 Ninth Avenue
Helena, MT 59620-0407
Telephone: 1-406-444-4284

Nebraska Board of Examiners in
Medicine and Surgery
P.O. Box 95007
Lincoln, NE 68509
Telephone: 1-402-471-2115

Nevada Board of Osteopathic
Examiners
1198 Sweetwater Drive
Reno, NV 89509
Telephone: 1-702-826-8383

New Hampshire Board of
Registration in Medicine
Health and Welfare Building
Hazen Drive
Concord, NH 03301
Telephone: 1-603-271-1203

New Jersey Board of Medical
Examiners
28 W. State Street
Room 602
Trenton, NJ 08608
Telephone: 1-609-292-4843

New Mexico Board of Osteopathic
Medical Examiners
725 St. Michaels Drive
P.O. Box 25101
Santa Fe, NM 87504
Telephone: 1-505-827-7171

New York Board for Medicine
Cultural Education Center
New York State Plaza
Room 3023
Albany, NY 12230
Telephone: 1-518-474-3841

North Carolina Board of Medical
Examiners
1313 Navaho Drive
Raleigh, NC 27609
Telephone: 1-919-876-3885

North Dakota Board of Medical
Examiners
418 E. Broad Way
City Center Plaza
Suite C-10
Bismarck, ND 58501
Telephone: 1-701-223-9485

Ohio State Medical Board
77 S. High Street, 17th Floor
Columbus, OH 43266-0315
Telephone: 1-614-466-3934

Oklahoma Board of Osteopathic
Examiners
4848 N. Lincoln Boulevard
Suite 100
Oklahoma City, OK 73105
Telephone: 1-405-528-8625

Oregon State Board of Medical
Examiners
1500 S.W. 1st Avenue
Room 620
Portland, OR 97201
Telephone: 1-503-229-5770

Pennsylvania Board of
Osteopathic Medical Examiners
P.O. Box 2649
Harrisburg, PA 17105
Telephone: 1-717-783-7156

Rhode Island Board of Medical
Licensure and Discipline
Department of Health
Cannon Building, Room 205
3 Capitol Hill
Providence, RI 20908-5097
Telephone: 1-401-277-3855

South Carolina Board of Medical
Examiners
1220 Pickens Street
Columbia, SC 29201
Telephone: 1-803-734-8901

South Dakota Board of Medical
and Osteopathic Examiners
1323 S. Minnesota Avenue
Sioux Falls, SD 57105
Telephone: 1-605-336-1965

Tennessee Board of Osteopathic
  Examination
283 Plus Park Boulevard
Nashville, TN 37219-5407
Telephone: 1-615-367-6393

Texas Board of Medical Examiners
P.O. Box 13562
Capitol Station
Austin, TX 78711
Telephone: 1-512-452-1078

Utah Department of Commerce
Division of Occupational and
  Professional Licensure
160 E. 300 South
P.O. Box 45802
Salt Lake City, UT 84145-0802
Telephone: 1-801-530-6628

Vermont Board of Osteopathic
  Examination and Registration
Secretary of State's Office
Pavilion Office Building
Montpelier, VT 05602
Telephone: 1-802-828-2673

Virginia State Board of Medicine
Department of Health
  Professionals
1601 Rolling Hills Drive
Richmond, VA 23229-5005
Telephone: 1-804-662-9908

Washington Division of
  Professional Licensing
P.O. Box 9012
Olympia, WA 98504
Telephone: 1-206-753-3095

West Virginia Board of Osteopathy
334 Penco Road
Weirton, WV 26062
Telephone: 1-304-723-4638

Wisconsin Medical Examining
  Board
P.O. Box 8935
Madison, WI 53708
Telephone: 1-608-266-2811

Wyoming Board of Medical
  Examiners
Barrett Building, 3d Floor
Cheyenne, WY 82002
Telephone: 1-307-777-6463

191

Appendix D

Licensing Boards *(Nursing)*

Alabama Board of Nursing
Attn: Legal Division
500 East Boulevard, Suite 203
1 East Building
Montgomery, AL 36117
Telephone: 1-205-261-4060

Alaska Division of Occupational
Licensing
3601 C Street, Suite 722
Anchorage, AK 99503
Telephone: 1-907-561-2878

Arizona Board of Nursing
2001 West Camelback, Suite 350
Phoenix, AZ 85015
Telephone: 1-602-255-5092

Arkansas Board of Nursing
Tower Building
1123 S. University, Suite 800
Little Rock, AR 72204
Telephone: 1-501-371-2751

California Board of Registered
Nursing
1030 13th Street
Room 200
Sacramento, CA 95814
Telephone: 1-916-322-3350

Colorado Board of Nursing
1560 Broadway, Suite 670
Denver, CO 80203
Telephone: 1-303-894-2430

Connecticut Board of Examiners
for Nursing
Public Health Hearing Office
150 W. Washington Street
Hartford, CT 06106
Telephone: 1-203-566-1011

Delaware Board of Nursing
Margaret O'Neill Building
P.O. Box 1401
Dover, DE 19903
Telephone: 1-302-736-4522

District of Columbia Department
of Consumer and Regulatory
Affairs
Attn: Complaint Division
614 H Street, N.W., Room 104
Washington, DC 20001
Telephone: 1-202-727-7107

Florida Department of Professional
Regulation
1940 N. Monroe Street
Tallahassee, FL 32399-0750
Telephone: 1-904-487-2252

Georgia Board of Nursing
166 Pryor Street, S.W.
Atlanta, GA 30303
Telephone: 1-404-656-3943

Hawaii Board of Nursing
P.O. Box 3469
Honolulu, HI 96801
Telephone: 1-808-548-3086

Idaho Board of Nursing
500 S. 10th, Suite 102
Boise, ID 83720
Telephone: 1-208-334-3110

Illinois Nursing Committee
Department of Registration and
   Education
320 W. Washington Street
Springfield, IL 62786
Telephone: 1-217-782-7116

Indiana Consumer Protection
   Division
219 State House
Indianapolis, IN 46204
Telephone: 1-317-232-6330;
   1-800-382-5516

Iowa Board of Nursing
1223 E. Court Avenue
Des Moines, IA 50319
Telephone: 1-515-281-3255

Kansas Board of Nursing
900 S.W. Jackson, Suite 551-S
Topeka, KS 66612-1256
Telephone: 1-913-296-4929

Kentucky Board of Nursing
4010 Dupont Circle, Suite 430
Louisville, KY 40207
Telephone: 1-502-897-5143

Louisiana Board of Nursing
907 Pere Marquette Building
150 Baronne Street
New Orleans, LA 70112
Telephone: 1-504-568-5464

Maine Board of Nursing
295 Water Street
Augusta, ME 04330
Telephone: 1-207-289-5324

Maryland Board of Nursing
4201 Patterson Avenue
Baltimore, MD 21215
Telephone: 1-301-764-4747

Massachusetts Board of
   Registration in Nursing
100 Cambridge Street
15th Floor
Boston, MA 02202
Telephone: 1-617-727-9961

Michigan Board of Nursing
Department of Licensing and
   Regulation
North Ottawa Tower Building
611 W. Ottawa
P.O. Box 30193
Lansing, MI 48909
Telephone: 1-517-373-1600

Minnesota Board of Nursing
2700 University Avenue, West
#108
St. Paul, MN 55114
Telephone: 1-612-642-0552

Mississippi Board of Nursing
239 N. Lamar Street
Suite 401
Jackson, MS 39201
Telephone: 1-601-359-6170

Missouri State Board of Nursing
P.O. Box 656
Jefferson City, MO 65102
Telephone: 1-314-751-2334

Montana Board of Nursing
Department of Commerce
1424 Ninth Avenue
Helena, MT 59620-0407
Telephone: 1-406-444-4279

Nebraska Bureau of Examining
   Boards
Nebraska Department of Health
301 Centennial Mall, South
Lincoln, NE 68509-5007
Telephone: 1-402-471-4921

Nevada Board of Nursing
1281 Terminal Way
Room 116
Reno, NV 89502
Telephone: 1-702-786-2778

New Hampshire Nurses
Registration Board
Division of Public Health
Health and Welfare Building
6 Hazen Drive
Concord, NH 03301-6527
Telephone: 1-603-271-2323

New Jersey Board of Nursing
1100 Raymond Boulevard
Room 508
Newark, NJ 07102
Telephone: 1-201-648-2570

New Mexico Board of Nursing
4125 Carlisle, N.E.
Albuquerque, NM 87107
Telephone: 1-505-841-6314

New York State Education
Department
Office of Professional Discipline
622 Third Avenue, 37th Floor
New York, NY 10017
Telephone: 1-212-557-2100;
1-800-422-8106

North Carolina Board of Nursing
P.O. Box 2129
Raleigh, NC 27602-2129
Telephone: 1-919-782-3211

North Dakota Board of Nursing
919 S. 7th Street
Suite 504
Bismarck, ND 58504
Telephone: 1-701-224-2974

Ohio Board of Nursing
77 S. High Street, 17th Floor
Columbus, OH 43266-0316
Telephone: 1-614-466-3947

Oklahoma Board of Nurse
Registration and Nursing
Education
2915 N. Classen Boulevard
Suite 524
Oklahoma City, OK 73106
Telephone: 1-405-525-2076

Oregon Board of Nursing
1400 S.W. 5th Avenue
Room 904
Portland, OR 97201
Telephone: 1-503-229-5653

Pennsylvania Bureau of
Professional and Occupational
Affairs
P.O. Box 2649
Harrisburg, PA 17105-2649
Telephone: 1-717-787-8503;
1-800-822-2113

Puerto Rico Office of Regulation
and Certification of Health
Professionals
Call Box 10200
Santurce, PR 00908
Telephone: 1-809-725-7506

Rhode Island Board of Nursing
Registration and Nursing
3 Capitol Hill
Providence, RI 02908
Telephone: 1-401-277-2827

South Carolina Board of Nursing
1777 St. Julian Place
Suite 102
Columbia, SC 29204-2488
Telephone: 1-803-737-6596

South Dakota Board of Nursing
304 S. Phillips Avenue
Suite 205
Sioux Falls, SD 57102
Telephone: 1-605-335-4973

Tennessee Board of Nursing
283 Plus Park Boulevard
Nashville, TN 37219-5407
Telephone: 1-615-367-6232

Texas Board of Nurse Examiners
9101 Burnet Road
Suite 104
Box 140466
Austin, TX 78714
Telephone: 1-512-835-4880

Utah Department of Occupational
and Professional Licensing
P.O. Box 45802
Salt Lake City, UT 84145
Telephone: 1-801-530-6628

Vermont Board of Nursing
26 Terrace Street
Montpelier, VT 05602
Telephone: 1-802-828-2396

Virgin Islands Department of
Health
Board of Nursing Licensing
P.O. Box 7309
St. Thomas, VI 00801
Telephone: 1-809-776-7397

Virginia Board of Nursing
Health Regulatory Board
Enforcement Division
1601 Rolling Hills Drive
Richmond, VA 23229-5005
Telephone: 1-804-662-9909;
1-800-533-1560

Washington Department of
Licensing
Nursing Board Professional
Program
Management Division
P.O. Box 9012
Olympia, WA 98504-8001
Telephone: 1-206-753-3726

West Virginia Board of Examiners
for Registered Nurses
922 Quarrier Street
Embleton Building, Suite 309
Charleston, WV 25301
Telephone: 1-304-348-3728

Wisconsin Department of
Licensing
Board of Nursing
P.O. Box 8935
Madison, WI 53708-8935
Telephone: 1-608-266-3735

Wyoming State Board of Nursing
Barrett Building, 3d Floor
2301 Central Avenue
Cheyenne, WY 82002
Telephone: 1-307-777-7601

Appendix E

Alabama Department of Public
Health
State Office Building
501 Dexter Avenue
Mail to: 434 Monroe Street
Montgomery, AL 36130-1701
Telephone: 1-205-242-5095

Alaska Department of Health and
Social Services
Alaska Office Building, Room 503
350 Main Street
Mail to: Pouch H-06
Juneau, AK 99811-0610
Telephone: 1-907-465-3030

Arizona Department of Health
Services
1740 W. Adams Street
Phoenix, AZ 85007
Telephone: 1-602-542-1024

Arkansas Department of Health
State Health Building
4815 W. Markham Street
Little Rock, AR 72205-3867
Telephone: 1-501-661-2112

California Department of Health
Services
714 P Street, Room 1253
Sacramento, CA 95814
Telephone: 1-916-445-1248

Colorado Department of Health
4210 E. 11th Avenue
Denver, CO 80220
Telephone: 1-303-331-4602

Connecticut Department of Health
Services
150 Washington Street
Hartford, CT 06106
Telephone: 1-203-566-2038

Delaware Division of Public Health
Department of Health and Social
Services
Jessie S. Cooper Building
Mail to: P.O. Box 637
Dover, DE 19901
Telephone: 1-302-736-4701

District of Columbia Department
of Human Services
Commission of Public Health
1660 L Street, N.W., 12th Floor
Washington, DC 20036
Telephone: 1-202-673-7700

Florida Health Program Office
Department of Health and
Rehabilitative Services
Building I, Room 115
1323 Winewood Boulevard
Tallahassee, FL 32399-0700
Telephone: 1-904-488-4115

Georgia Division of Public Health
Department of Human Resources
878 Peachtree Street, N.E.
Suite 201
Atlanta, GA 30309
Telephone: 1-404-894-7505

Hawaii Department of Health
Kinau Hale
1250 Punchbowl Street
Mail to: P.O. Box 3378
Honolulu, HI 96801
Telephone: 1-808-548-6505

Idaho Bureau of Preventive
Medicine
Division of Health
Department of Health and Welfare
Towers Building, 4th Floor
450 W. State Street
Boise, ID 83720
Telephone: 1-208-334-5930

Illinois Department of Public
Health
535 W. Jefferson Street
Springfield, IL 62761
Telephone: 1-217-782-4977

Indiana State Board of Health
1330 W. Michigan Street
Mail to: P.O. Box 1964
Indianapolis, IN 46206-1964
Telephone: 1-317-633-8400

Iowa Department of Public Health
Lucas State Office Building
E. 12th and Walnut Streets
Des Moines, IA 50319
Telephone: 1-515-281-5605

Kansas Division of Health
Department of Health and
Environment
Building 740
Forbes Field
Topeka, KS 66620
Telephone: 1-913-296-1500

Kentucky Department for Health
Services
Cabinet for Human Resources
Health Services Building, 1st
Floor
275 E. Main Street
Frankfort, KY 40621
Telephone: 1-502-564-3970

Louisiana Department of
Hospitals DHH
Office of Public Health Services
325 Loyola Avenue
Mail to: P.O. Box 60630
New Orleans, LA 70160
Telephone: 1-504-568-5052

Maine Bureau of Health
Department of Human Services
157 Capitol Street
Mail to: State House, Station 11
Augusta, ME 04333
Telephone: 1-207-289-3201

Maryland Department of Health
and Mental Hygiene
Herbert R. O'Conor State Office
Building
201 W. Preston Street
Baltimore, MD 21201
Telephone: 1-301-225-6500

Massachusetts Department of
Public Health
150 Tremont Street
Boston, MA 02111
Telephone: 1-617-727-0201

Michigan Department of Public
Health
Baker-Olin West Building
3423 N. Logan Street
Mail to: P.O. Box 30195
Lansing, MI 48909
Telephone: 1-517-335-8000

Minnesota Department of Health
717 Delaware Street, S.E.
Mail to: P.O. Box 9441
Minneapolis, MN 55440
Telephone: 1-612-623-5460

Mississippi Department of Health
2423 N. State Street
Mail to: P.O. Box 1700
Jackson, MS 39215-1700
Telephone: 1-601-960-7400

Missouri Department of Health
Mail to: P.O. Box 570
Jefferson City, MO 65102
Telephone: 1-314-751-6001

Montana Department of Health
and Environmental Sciences
Cogswell Building, Room C108
Helena, MT 59620
Telephone: 1-406-444-2544

Nebraska Department of Health
State Office Building
301 Centennial Mall, South
Mail to: P.O. Box 95007
Lincoln, NE 68509
Telephone: 1-402-471-2133

Nevada Health Division
Department of Human Resources
Kinkead Building
505 E. King Street
Mail to: Capitol Complex
Carson City, NV 89710
Telephone: 1-702-885-4740

New Hampshire Division of Public
Health Services
Department of Health & Human
Services
Health and Welfare Services
Building
6 Hazen Drive
Concord, NH 03301-6527
Telephone: 1-603-271-4501

New Jersey Department of Health
Health and Agriculture Building
John Fitch Plaza
Mail to: CN 360
Trenton, NJ 08625
Telephone: 1-609-292-7837

New Mexico Division of Public
Health
Health and Environment
Department
Harold Runnels Building
1190 St. Francis Drive
Santa Fe, NM 87503
Telephone: 1-505-827-0020

New York Department of Health
Corning Tower, Room 1408
Empire State Plaza
Albany, NY 12237
Telephone: 1-518-474-2011

North Carolina Department of
Environment, Health and Natural
Resources
Office of the State Health Director
Archdale Building
512 N. Salisbury Street
Mail to: P.O. Box 27687
Raleigh, NC 27611
Telephone: 1-919-733-3446

North Dakota Department of
Health
State Capitol
600 E. Boulevard Avenue
Bismarck, ND 58505-0200
Telephone: 1-701-224-2372

Ohio Department of Health
246 N. High Street
Columbus, OH 43226-0588
Telephone: 1-614-466-3543

Oklahoma Department of Health
1000 N.E. 10th Street
Mail to: P.O. Box 53551
Oklahoma City, OK 73152
Telephone: 1-405-271-4200

Oregon Health Division
Department of Human Resources
State Office Building, Room 811
1400 S.W. 5th Avenue
Mail to: P.O. Box 231
Portland, OR 97207
Telephone: 1-503-229-5032

Pennsylvania Department of
Health
Health and Welfare Building,
Room 802
Commonwealth Avenue and
Forster Street
Mail to: P.O. Box 90
Harrisburg, PA 17108
Telephone: 1-717-787-6436

Puerto Rico Department of Health
Call Box 70184
San Juan, PR 00936
Telephone: 1-809-250-7227

Rhode Island Department of
Health
Cannon Building, Room 401
Three Capitol Hill
Providence, RI 02908
Telephone: 1-401-277-2231

South Carolina Department of
Health and Environmental
Control
2600 Bull Street
Columbia, SC 29201
Telephone: 1-803-734-4880

South Dakota Department of
Health
Joe Foss Building
523 E. Capitol Avenue
Pierre, SD 57501
Telephone: 1-605-773-3361

Tennessee Department of Health
and Environment
Cordell Hull Building
Room 344
Nashville, TN 37219
Telephone: 1-615-741-3111

Texas Department of Health
1100 W. 49th Street
Austin, TX 78756-3199
Telephone: 1-512-458-7375

Utah Department of Health
288 N. 1460 West
Salt Lake City, UT 84116-0700
Telephone: 1-801-538-6101

Vermont Department of Health
Agency of Human Services
60 Main Street
Mail to: P.O. Box 70
Burlington, VT 05402
Telephone: 1-802-863-7280

Virgin Islands Department of
Health
St. Thomas Hospital
Charlotte Amalie
St. Thomas, VI 00802
Telephone: 1-809-774-0117

Virginia Department of Health
James Madison Building
109 Governor Street
Richmond, VA 23219
Telephone: 1-804-786-3561

Washington Division of Health
Department of Health
1112 S. Quince Street
Mail to: Mail Stop ET-21
Olympia, WA 98504
Telephone: 1-206-753-5871

West Virginia Department of
Health
State Office Building 3, Room 206
1800 Washington Street, E.
Charleston, WV 25305
Telephone: 1-304-348-2971

Wisconsin Division of Health
Department of Health and Social
Services
Mail to: P.O. Box 309
Madison, WI 53701-0309
Telephone: 1-608-266-7568

Wyoming Department of Health
and Social Services
Hathaway Building
2300 Capitol Avenue
Cheyenne, WY 82002-0710
Telephone: 1-307-777-7656

The two lists below do not represent an "Either-Or" situation. Most parents choose their options from both pathways. Very few doctors or midwives practice completely in accordance with either pathway. Consider and discuss each option and then decide which you prefer. Flexibility is necessary to ensure that the Birth Plan will apply in difficult or complicated labors as well as normal and typical labors.

Medical Pathway	Physiologic Pathway

(Which of these are routines and which are options in your hospital or birth center? Most parents choose some options from each list.)

Labor

Medical Pathway	Physiologic Pathway
· Mother in wheelchair upon arrival at hospital.	· Mother walks to labor and delivery.
· Shave, minishave, or clipping of long hairs on perineum.	· No shave or clipping of hair.
· Enema.	· Bowels emptied spontaneously, or enema self-administered at home.
· Partner is asked to leave during prep and exams.	· Partner present throughout labor and delivery.
· Limit to one support person during labor and birth.	· Presence of other friends, relatives, and siblings.
· Confinement to bed and/or one position.	· Freedom to walk and change positions as desired.
· Induction of labor.	· Spontaneous Labor.
· Methods: Stripping membranes, amniotomy, oxytocin.	Alternatives: Making love, breast stimulation.
· IV fluids for hydration and energy.	· Drinking fluid or eating as desired.
· Frequent vaginal exams.	· Vaginal exams when requested by mother or for medical reasons.
· Electronic Fetal Heart Monitor.	· Listening to fetal heart with fetal stethoscope.
· Pain Relief through medication: analgesics or anesthetics.	· Relaxation, emotional support, massage, breathing.

Birth

Medical Pathway	Physiologic Pathway
· Lithotomy position or semisitting in labor bed for pushing.	· Choice of position and freedom to move.
· Prolonged breathholding and bearing down for expulsion.	· Mother follows her urge to push.
· Limit of two hours on 2d stage—then forceps or cesarean birth.	· Allow for longer 2d stage and position variations to help progress.
· Delivery table for birth.	· Birth in labor bed, birth chair, or bean bag.
· Lithotomy position with stirrups for birth.	· Sidelying, all fours, squatting, standing with leg up, semireclining with back support, no stirrups.
· Mother not allowed to touch sterile field.	· Mother allowed to touch baby's head as it crowns.
· Catheterization in second stage.	· No catheterization and frequent voiding in first stage.
· Episiotomy.	· No episiotomy: massage, warm compresses, slower delivery, coaching to pant out baby, support to perineum.
	Late episiotomy with no anesthesia.
· Forceps or vacuum extraction.	· Spontaneous delivery.

After Birth

Medical Pathway	Physiologic Pathway
· Intubation/Suctioning.	· Waiting to see if baby can handle own mucus.
· Immediate care of baby done out of sight of mother: e.g., identification, Apgar, heat lamp, replace hemostat with cord clamp.	· Care done on mother's abdomen. Baby skin to skin with mother with heat lamp or blanket over them.
	Delay in nonessential routines.

- Limit of 15–20 minutes on 3d stage followed by manual extraction of the placenta.
- Pitocin drip or injection for contraction of uterus after placenta is born.

- Allow for longer time for placenta. Allow mother to move around, nurse baby. Let cord drain.
- Evaluation of uterus before using uterine stimulant routinely. Breast-feeding.

Baby

- Baby to isolette or nursery for 4–24 hours. Mother to recovery room for observation.
- Eye drops—silver nitrate applied shortly after birth.
- Baby's first feeding—glucose water by nurse.
- Baby in nursery except for scheduled 4-hour feedings.
- Circumcision.
- Home in 3 or more days after delivery.

- Baby held by mother or father on delivery table and/or in recovery.
- Omit eye drops or delay administration up to 2 hours. Use of other agent as alternative.
- Colostrum by mother who plans to breast-feed or plain water given by mother.
- Demand feeding, baby to mother when crying. Twenty-four-hour rooming-in.
- No circumcision.
- Parents present to comfort baby after operation.
- Early discharge from hospital.

Cesarean Birth

THE UNEXPECTED

Common Medical Procedures

- Scheduled surgery.
- Mother without her support person in surgery.
- General anesthesia.
- Screen to prevent viewing surgery.

- Mother not allowed to wear contacts or glasses.
- Baby sent to Intensive Care Nursery.

Possible Options

- Surgery after labor begins.
- Father present to support mother.
- Spinal or epidural.
- Screen lowered at time of birth or baby held up for mother and father to see.
- Mother to wear contacts or glasses.
- Father to hold baby and mother to see baby, if baby is not in distress. Mother allowed to breast-feed in recovery if her and her baby's condition permit.

Premature Sick Infant

- Baby cared for by professionals.
- Baby rushed to intensive care.
- Baby sent to another hospital or another part of hospital.
- Baby transported to hospital with intensive care unit.
- Limited visits to baby from mother only.
- IV and bottle feeding.

- Parents involved in care of baby, diapering, touching, talking to baby in incubator, feeding baby.
- Mother allowed to hold and see baby, if not distressed.
- Baby close to mother; in same part of hospital.
- Father goes with the transport team, mother goes if she is able.
- Father and/or extended family allowed to see baby.
- Mother allowed to express her colostrum for the baby and encouraged and helped to get started at breast-feeding.

Appendix G

━━━━ *A Patient's Bill of Rights*

The American Hospital Association presents *A Patient's Bill of Rights* with the expectation that observance of these rights will contribute to more effective patient care and greater satisfaction for the patient, his physician, and the hospital organization. Further, the association presents these rights in the expectation that they will be supported by the hospital on behalf of its patients as an integral part of the healing process. It is recognized that a personal relationship between the physician and the patient is essential for the provision of proper medical care.

The traditional physician-patient relationship takes on a new dimension when care is rendered within an organizational structure. Legal precedent has established that the institution itself also has a responsibility to the patient. It is in recognition of these factors that these rights are affirmed.

1. The patient has the right to considerate and respectful care.

2. The patient has the right to obtain from his physician complete current information concerning his diagnosis, treatment, and prognosis in terms the patient can be reasonably expected to understand. When it is not medically advisable to give such information to the patient, the information should be made available to an appropriate person in his behalf. He

203

has the right to know, by name, the physician responsible for coordinating his care.

3. The patient has the right to receive from his physician information necessary to give informed consent prior to the start of any procedure and/or treatment. Except in emergencies, such information for informed consent should include, but not necessarily be limited to, the specific procedure and/or treatment, the medically significant risks involved, and the probable duration of incapacitation. Where medically significant alternatives for care or treatment exist, or when the patient requests information concerning medical alternatives, the patient has the right to such information. The patient also has the right to know the name of the person responsible for the procedures and/or treatment.

4. The patient has the right to refuse treatment to the extent permitted by law and to be informed of the medical consequences of his action.

5. The patient has the right to every consideration of his privacy concerning his own medical care program. Case discussion, consultation, examination, and treatment are confidential and should be conducted discreetly. Those not directly involved in his care must have the permission of the patient to be present.

6. The patient has the right to expect that all communications and records pertaining to his care should be treated as confidential.

7. The patient has the right to expect that within its capacity a hospital must make reasonable response to the request of a patient for services. The hospital must provide evaluation, service, and/or referral as indicated by the urgency of the case. When medically permissible, a patient may be transferred to another facility only after he has received complete information and explanation concerning the needs for and alternatives to such a transfer. The institution to which the patient is to be transferred must first have accepted the patient for transfer.

8. The patient has the right to obtain information as to any relationship of his hospital to other health care and educational institutions insofar as his care is concerned. The patient has the right to obtain information as to the existence of any

professional relationships among the individuals, by name, who are treating him.

9. The patient has the right to be advised if the hospital proposes to engage in or perform human experimentation affecting his care or treatment. The patient has the right to refuse to participate in such research projects.

10. The patient has the right to expect reasonable continuity of care. He has the right to know in advance what appointment times and physicians are available and where. The patient has the right to expect that the hospital will provide a mechanism whereby he is informed by his physician or a delegate of the physician of the patient's continuing health care requirements following discharge.

11. The patient has the right to examine and receive an explanation of his bill, regardless of source of payment.

12. The patient has the right to know what hospital rules and regulations apply to his conduct as a patient.

Appendix H

────── *Pregnant Patient's Bill of Rights and Responsibilities*

1. The Pregnant Patient has the right, prior to the administration of any drug or procedure, to be informed by the health professional caring for her of any potential direct or indirect effects, risks or hazards to herself or her unborn or newborn infant which may result from the use of a drug or procedure prescribed for or administered to her during pregnancy, labor, birth, or lactation.

2. The Pregnant Patient has the right, prior to the proposed therapy, to be informed, not only of the benefits, risks, and hazards of the proposed therapy but also of known alternative therapy, such as available childbirth education classes which could help to prepare the Pregnant Patient physically and mentally to cope with the discomfort or stress of pregnancy and the experience of childbirth, thereby reducing or eliminating her need for drugs and obstetric intervention. She should be offered such information early in her pregnancy in order that she may make a reasoned decision.

3. The Pregnant Patient has the right, prior to the administration of any drug, to be informed by the health professional who is prescribing or administering the drug to her that any drug which she receives during pregnancy, labor and birth, no matter how or when the drug is taken or administered, may

adversely affect her unborn baby, directly or indirectly, and that there is no drug or chemical which has been proven safe for the unborn child.

4. The Pregnant Patient has the right, if cesarean section is anticipated, to be informed prior to the administration of any drug, and preferably prior to her hospitalization, that minimizing her and, in turn, her baby's intake of nonessential preoperative medicine will benefit her baby.

5. The Pregnant Patient has the right, prior to the administration of a drug or procedure, to be informed of the areas of uncertainty if there is NO properly controlled follow-up research which has established the safety of the drug or procedure with regard to its direct and/or indirect effects on the physiological, mental and neurological development of the child exposed, via the mother, to the drug or procedure during pregnancy, labor, birth, or lactation (this would apply to virtually all drugs and the vast majority of obstetric procedures).

6. The Pregnant Patient has the right, prior to the administration of any drug, to be informed of the brand name and generic name of the drug in order that she may advise the health professional of any past adverse reaction to the drug.

7. The Pregnant Patient has the right to determine for herself, without pressure from the attendant, whether she will accept the risks inherent in the proposed therapy or refuse a drug or procedure.

8. The Pregnant Patient has the right to know the name and qualifications of the individual administering a medication or procedure to her during labor or birth.

9. The Pregnant Patient has the right to be informed, prior to the administration of any procedure, whether that procedure is being administered to her for her or her baby's benefit (medically indicated) or as an elective procedure (for convenience, teaching purposes, or research).

10. The Pregnant Patient has the right to be accompanied during the stress of labor and birth by someone she cares for, and to whom she looks for emotional comfort and encouragement.

11. The Pregnant Patient has the right after appropriate med-

ical consultation to choose a position for labor and for birth which is least stressful to her baby and to herself.

12. The Obstetric Patient has the right to have her baby cared for at her bedside if the baby is normal, and to feed her baby according to her baby's needs rather than according to the hospital regimen.

13. The Obstetric Patient has the right to be informed in writing of the name of the person who actually delivered her baby and the professional qualifications of that person. This information should also be on the birth certificate.

14. The Obstetric Patient has the right to be informed if there is any known or indicated aspect of her baby's care or condition which may cause her or her baby later difficulty or problems.

15. The Obstetric Patient has the right to have her and her baby's hospital medical records complete, accurate and legible and to have their records, including nursing notes, and to receive a copy upon payment of a reasonable fee and without incurring the expense of retaining an attorney.

16. The Obstetric Patient, both during and after her hospital stay, has the right to have access to her complete hospital medical records, including nursing notes, and to receive a copy upon payment of a reasonable fee and without incurring the expense of retaining an attorney.

1. The Pregnant Patient is responsible for learning about the physical and psychological process of labor, birth, and post-partum recovery. The better informed expectant parents are, the better they will be able to participate in decisions concerning the planning of their care.

2. The Pregnant Patient is responsible for learning what comprises good prenatal and intranatal care and for making an effort to obtain the best care possible.

3. Expectant parents are responsible for knowing about those hospital policies and regulations which will affect their birth and postpartum experience.

4. The Pregnant Patient is responsible for arranging for a companion or support person (husband, mother, sister, friend,

etc.) who will share in her plans for birth and who will accompany her during her labor and birth experience.

5. The Pregnant Patient is responsible for making her preferences known clearly to the health professional involved in her case in a courteous and cooperative manner and for making mutually agreed upon arrangements regarding maternity care alternatives with her physician or hospital in advance of labor.

6. Expectant parents are responsible for listening to their chosen physician or midwife with an open mind, just as they expect him or her to listen openly to them.

7. Once they have agreed to a course of health care, expectant parents are responsible, to the best of their ability, for seeing that the program is carried out in consultation with others with whom they have made the agreement.

8. The Pregnant Patient is responsible for obtaining information in advance regarding the approximate cost of her obstetric and hospital care.

9. The Pregnant Patient who intends to change her physician or hospital is responsible for notifying all concerned, well in advance of the birth if possible, and for informing both of her reasons for changing.

10. In all their interactions with medical and nursing personnel, the expectant parents should behave toward those caring for them with the same respect and consideration they themselves would like.

11. During the mother's hospital stay, the mother is responsible for learning about her and her baby's continuing care after discharge from the hospital.

12. After birth, the parents should put into writing constructive comments and feelings of satisfaction and/or dissatisfaction with the care (nursing, medical, and personal) they received. Good service to families in the future will be facilitated by those parents who take the time and responsibility to write letters expressing their feelings about the maternity care they received.

Source: International Childbirth Education Association, P.O. Box 20048, Minneapolis, MN 55420

Appendix I

——— *Where to Go for Help*

A.M.E.N.D. (Aiding Mothers and Fathers Experiencing Neonatal Death)
c/o Maureen Connelly
4324 Berrywick Terrace
St. Louis, Missouri 63128
Telephone: 1-314-487-7582

American Academy of Husband-Coached Childbirth
P.O. Box 5224
Sherman Oaks, California 91413-5224
Telephone: 1-800-42-BIRTH (in California); 1-800-423-3297; 1-818-788-6662

American Board of Family Practice
2228 Young Drive
Lexington, Kentucky 40505
Telephone: 1-606-269-5626

American Board of Internal Medicine
University City Science Center
3624 Market Street
Philadelphia, Pennsylvania 19104
Telephone: 1-215-243-1500

American Board of Medical Genetics
9650 Rockville Pike
Bethesda, Maryland 20814
Telephone: 1-301-571-1825

American Board of Obstetrics and Gynecology
4225 Roosevelt Way, N.E., Suite 305
Seattle, Washington 98105
Telephone: 1-206-547-4884

American Board of Urology
31700 Telegraph Road, Suite 150
Birmingham, Michigan 48010
Telephone: 1-313-646-9720

American College of Home Obstetrics
P.O. Box 508
Oak Park, Illinois 60303
Telephone: 1-708-383-1461
The college was founded to bring together those physicians who wish to cooperate with families who choose to give birth in the home. In response to inquiries, it will furnish the names of doctors (if any) in the area who will attend home births.

American College of Nurse-
Midwives
1522 K Street, N.W., Suite 1000
Washington, D.C. 20005
Telephone: 1-202-289-4379

American College of Obstetricians
and Gynecologists
409 12th Street, S.W.
Washington, D.C. 20024-2188
Telephone: 1-202-638-5577

American Fertility Society
2140 11th Avenue South, Suite
200
Birmingham, Alabama 35205-
2800
Telephone: 1-205-933-8494

American Osteopathic Board of
General Practice
330 E. Algonquin Road, #2
Arlington Heights, Illinois 60005
Telephone: 1-708-635-8477

American Osteopathic Board of
Obstetrics and Gynecology
5200 S. Ellis Street
Chicago, Illinois 60615
Telephone: 1-312-947-3000

American Society for
Psychoprophylaxis in Obstetrics/
Lamaze
1101 Connecticut Avenue, N.W.,
Suite 300
Washington, D.C. 20036
Telephone: 1-202-857-1128

Barren Foundation, The
65 E. Wacker Place, Suite 2408
Chicago, Illinois 60601
Telephone: 1-312-782-1356
The Barren Foundation is an organization dedicated to research and
public education in the field of reproductive endocrinology. Its services include support groups, medical seminars, and literature on
infertility.

Boston Women's Health Book
Collective
Box 192
West Somerville, Massachusetts
02144
Telephone: 1-617-625-0271

Boston Women's Health
Information Center
240A Elm Street, 3d floor (Davis
Square)
Somerville, Massachusetts 02144
Telephone: 1-617-625-0271

Center for Study of Multiple Birth
333 Superior Street, Suite 476
Chicago, Illinois 60611
Telephone: 1-312-266-9093

Center for Surrogate Parenting
8383 Wilshire Boulevard, Suite
750
Beverly Hills, California 90211
Telephone: 1-213-655-1974

Cesarean Prevention Movement
P.O. Box 152
University Station
Syracuse, New York 13210
Telephone: 1-315-424-1942

Cesarean/Support, Education and
Concern, Inc. (C/SEC, Inc.)
10 Speen Street
Framingham, Massachusetts
01701
Telephone: 1-508-820-2760

Compassionate Friends
P.O. Box 3696
Oak Brook, Illinois 60522-3696
Telephone: 1-708-990-0010
This national organization (six
hundred chapters) offers support to
parents and siblings bereaving the
death of a child.

DES Action
1615 Broadway, #510
Oakland, California 94612
Telephone: 1-415-465-4011

Farm Midwifery Center, The
48 The Farm
Summertown, Tennessee 38483
Telephone: 1-615-964-2293
Operating for more than twenty
years in rural Tennessee, The Farm
has a national reputation in home
birth and the practice of empirical
midwifery. In addition to complete
maternity care, parent classes,
breast-feeding counseling, and library services are available.

International Childbirth Education
Association
P.O. Box 20048
Minneapolis, Minnesota 55420
Telephone: 1-612-854-8660

Joint Commission on Accreditation
of Healthcare Organizations
1 Renaissance Boulevard
Oakbrook Terrace, Illinois 60181
Telephone: 1-708-916-5600

La Leche League International
9616 Minneapolis Avenue
P.O. Box 1209
Franklin Park, Illinois 60131-
8209
Telephone: 1-708-455-7730

March of Dimes Birth Defects
Foundation
1275 Mamaroneck Avenue
White Plains, New York 10605
Telephone: 1-914-428-7100

Maternal and Child Health Center
2464 Massachusetts Avenue
Cambridge, Massachusetts 02140
Telephone: 1-617-864-9343

Maternity Center Association
48 E. 92d Street
New York, New York 10128
Telephone: 1-212-369-7300

National Association of
Childbearing Centers
3123 Gottschall Road
Perkiomenville, Pennsylvania
18074
Telephone: 1-215-234-8068

National Association of Parents and
Professionals for Safe
Alternatives in Childbirth
Route 1, Box 646
Marble Hill, Missouri 63764
Telephone: 1-314-238-2010

National Association of Surrogate
Mothers
8383 Wilshire Boulevard, Suite
750
Beverly Hills, California 90211
Telephone: 1-213-655-2015

National Center for Education in
Maternal and Child Health
38th and R Streets, N.W.
Washington, D.C. 20057
Telephone: 1-202-625-8400

National Foundation for Jewish
Genetic Diseases
250 Park Avenue, Suite 1000
New York, New York 10177
Telephone: 1-212-371-1030

National Institute for Occupational
Safety and Health (NIOSH)
4676 Columbia Parkway
Cincinnati, Ohio 45226
Telephone: 1-800-356-4674

National Maternal and Child Health
Clearinghouse
38th and R Streets, N.W.
Washington, D.C. 20057
Telephone: 1-202-625-8410

Occupational Safety and Health
Administration
U.S. Department of Labor
200 Constitution Avenue, N.W.
Room 3647
Washington, D.C. 20210
Telephone: 1-202-523-8151
(Public and Consumer
Information)

Pennypress, Inc.
1100 23d Avenue East
Seattle, Washington 98112
Telephone: 1-206-325-1419
Pennypress is a woman-owned,
woman-run publisher of materials
on childbirth and parenting.

Planned Parenthood
  810 Seventh Avenue
  New York, New York 10019
  Telephone: 1-212-541-7800

Read Natural Childbirth
  Foundation, Inc.
  P.O. Box 150956
  San Rafael, California 94915
  Telephone: 1-415-456-8462

RESOLVE
  5 Water Street
  Arlington, Massachusetts 02174
  Telephone: 1-617-643-2424;
    1-800-662-1016

S.H.A.R.E. (Source of Help in
  Airing and Resolving
  Experiences)
  c/o St. Elizabeth's Hospital
  211 S. Third Street
  Belleville, Illinois 62222
  Telephone: 1-618-234-2415

Society of Assisted Reproductive
  Technology
  2140 11th Avenue South, Suite
    200
  Birmingham, Alabama 35205-
    2800
  Telephone: 1-205-933-8494

Surrogates by Choice
  P.O. Box 05257
  Detroit, Michigan 48205
  Telephone: 1-313-839-4946

Triplet Connection, The
  8900 Thornton Road, #25
  P.O. Box 99571
  Stockton, California 95209
  Telephone: 1-209-474-0885
The Triplet Connection is an orga-
nization for parents who have had a
multiple birth of three or more.

Twin Services
  P.O. Box 10066
  Berkeley, California 94709
  Telephone: 1-415-524-0863

Unite, Inc.
  c/o Janis Heil
  Jeanes Hospital
  7600 Central Avenue
  Philadelphia, Pennsylvania 19111
  Telephone: 1-215-728-2082 or
    728-3777
Unite offers support for parents
grieving miscarriage, stillbirth, and
infant death.

Index

221

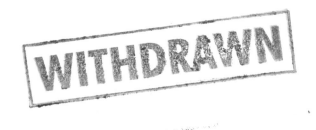